Advance F

MW00584383

"Colors of Hope provide
churches who long to
well as to LGBTQ+ folks who want to begin to integrate
gender identity, and spirituality. Reflecting on the colors of the Pride
flag, each contributor offers a reflection on the meaning from their
perspective and the chance for readers to embody the meaning
for themselves. There are still so few devotionals that are LGBTQ+
affirming, and this book is a welcome additional resource."
— **Fr. Shannon T.L. Kearns (he/him), co-founder,
QueerTheology.com and co-author of *Queers the Word***

"Colors of Hope will both settle and agitate your soul. A cadre of
spiritual leaders merge biblical stories and passages with the themes
of Gilbert Baker's rainbow Pride flag, giving a faithful weightiness
to the broad, diverse LGBTQ community. This book will move you
beyond pride, into a holistic understanding of who God made you to
be, and what you are called to do in the world."
— **Ross Murray (he/him), author, *Made, Known, Loved:
Developing LGBTQ-Inclusive Youth Ministry***

"The words of the Bible, in black and white, are often a source of
despair for LGBTQ+ people, but *Colors of Hope* presents a diverse
collection of writers who understand the hope embodied in both
scripture and the colors of the Pride flag. For too long, the LGBTQ+
community has been expected to confine their lives within the
constructs of traditional Christianity. Within the pages of this book,
however, the depth and beauty of LGBTQ+ spirituality, and how God
continually leads us to color outside the lines of tradition, bleed
through each page."
— **Candace Chellew (she/her), author, *Bulletproof Faith: A
Spiritual Survival Guide for Gay and Lesbian Christians* and
founder of *Whosoever: An Online Magazine for LGBTQ+
Christians***

"If you are looking for an easy-to-read and transformative devotional, you need *Colors of Hope*. This book amplifies unique voices that make us wonder, resist, embody, create, hope, stretch, and share in a way that is thought-provoking and contemporary. As I read the devotional, I found myself reflecting deeply on the journal prompts. Using the inclusive colors of the rainbow flag, we are offered a new way of seeing color in the world around us and allowed to reflect and write about our own experiences. As you travel through the book, allow yourself to be open to the world around you and the colors that may impact on the journey. *Colors of Hope* offers a connection to God, your faith, and your experience in order to live your authentic and whole self. A must-read for any pilgrim on the journey of love and hope."

— **Rev. Wanda Floyd (she/her), Founding Pastor, Imani MCC, Durham, NC, USA, and Emerging Church and MCC Communities Co-Ordinator for Metropolitan Community Churches**

"The gift of *Colors of Hope* to readers begins with the 'Acknowledgements' and moves with grace throughout the devotional journal's nine themes. This is a book that with each chapter and page does the radical and prophetic work of acknowledgment. It acknowledges that we are all God's beloved children. It acknowledges with hopeful and generous hospitality that each of our journeys into the love of God is unique and valuable. It acknowledges the voices of contributors who embody God's acknowledgment of each person's worth in their daily work as community leaders. In a world where too many people go unnoticed, unaccepted, and unrecognized—go unacknowledged— *Colors of Hope* offers words of care and an invitation to 'individually and collectively hope in color.'"

— **Jill Y. Crainshaw (she/her), Wake Forest University School of Divinity**

"*Colors of Hope* is a powerful, queer, adult 'coloring' book of the Spirit! The simplicity of using the colors of the Pride flag to inspire and ask fresh questions will be life changing for so many. I was so blessed by the diversity of voices. The rich particularity in the stories make this useful as well as transformative. *Colors of Hope is* a spirit-lifter for a community that really needs it in these times!"
— **Rev. Dr. Nancy Wilson (she/her), former global Moderator of Metropolitan Community Churches**

"It is rare I open a book and instantly feel hurt that I wasn't invited to add my own words. I was left asking myself a lot of questions: have I not been brave as these souls, have I not shined brightly enough? Have I not drenched my liturgies, love, culture, and liberation in enough glitter to be asked to join this particular endeavor? Empire is falling and sacred queer history, culture, worship, and theology is a precious jewel in an undeserving world. I pray this book leaves you like me, asking questions: am I willing to do my part in the Divine chain of queer saints, poets, mystics, and seekers knowing that I may lose or that I may fail? Do I truly know, like so many others before and all around me, that I will rise again, like the rainbow? Would I do it for brief moments of colorful explosions of Divine transition?"
— **Rev. Lenny Duncan (they/them), author, witness, agitator, PhD candidate**

COLORS
— OF —
HOPE

A DEVOTIONAL JOURNAL FROM
LGBTQ+ CHRISTIANS

MELISSA GUTHRIE, Editor

**chalice
press**

Saint Louis, Missouri

An imprint of Christian Board of Publication

New Revised Standard Version (NRSV)

The Message (Message)

New Living Translation (NLT)

Cover design: 99Designs

ChalicePress.com

Print: 9780827207479

EPUB: 9780827207486

EPDF: 9780827207493

Printed in the United States of America

This book is dedicated to three men who have always loved all of me.

My brother, Marc Robert Guthrie

My father, Robert Orie Guthrie

My stepfather, David "Dave" Hazen

My brother rises against life's challenges daily.
My father and stepfather rest eternally.

Contents

Contributors

Tyler Heston

Tyler Heston (he/him) is an ordained minister with the Christian Church (Disciples of Christ) living in Kansas City, Missouri, and serving at Country Club Christian Church. He believes that there is transformative power at the intersection of queerness and spirituality. Tyler, originally from Memphis, Tennessee, is a graduate of Brite Divinity School in Fort Worth, Texas, and enjoys things like *The X-Files*, niche pop music, and long hours journaling at the coffee shop.

Alysha Laperche

Alysha Laperche (they/them) holds a bachelor's degree in Social Work and a Master of Arts in Theology from Phillips Theological Seminary. They are grateful and excited for opportunities to continue following their call to embody the inclusive love of God revealed in Jesus Christ, particularly through working to actualize the vision of setting a place at the table for people of all sexual orientations and gender identities. Alysha is co-creator of the *Colors of Hope* podcast series with AllianceQ.

Sandhya Rani Jha

Sandhya Jha (she/they) is an anti-oppression consultant. Founder and former executive director of the Oakland Peace Center, Sandhya is comfortable in the pulpit, on the picket line, or hanging out with friends and friends-to-be over a good cup of tea and a good story. Sandhya is an ordained pastor in the Christian Church (Disciples of Christ). They are currently working on their fifth book for Chalice Press.

Nadia Tavera

Nadia Tavera (she/they) was born and raised in Mexico City. They graduated from Pacific School of Religion and is on the ordination track with the Disciples of Christ Northern California-Nevada Region. Nadia's calling is to minister with LGBTQ+ Latinx folks. She has a passion for accompanying people in their coming out process. Nadia believes that living in community is a meaningful way to experience God's love and a path to abundant life.

Andrew Deeb

Andy Deeb (he/him) is a born and raised Michigander. He is a PhD student in Bible and Cultures (Hebrew Bible) at Drew University. Andy is also a musician and worship leader who seeks to combine charismatic styles of worship with affirming theology. When not doing schoolwork or making music, he can usually be found playing video games or running.

William DeShay C. Jackson

DeShay Jackson (they/them) serves as Minister of Music for First Christian Church in Granbury, Texas. They hold a Master of Divinity from Brite Divinity School with certificates in Black Church Studies and Gender and Sexual Justice and a Bachelor of Music Education from Culver-Stockton College. DeShay is seeking ordination with the Mid-America region of the Christian Church. DeShay's interests center the importance of Womanism and its influence on Black/LGBTQIA+ culture, music, and food.

Melissa Guthrie

Melissa Lynn Guthrie (she/her) is the Executive Director + Minister with AllianceQ and the founding director of Salvage Garden. She created "The Banquet: A Sensory Worship Experience," centering disabled individuals. Melissa is trained in faith-based nonprofit leadership through Wake Forest University. A Wartburg College alumna (Waverly, Iowa), the Spirit moved Melissa to North Carolina to teach high school English as a corps member with Teach for America. Melissa and her wife Leah live in Greensboro, North Carolina, with their children and a small zoo.

Renair Amin

Dr. Renair Amin (she/they) is an author, international speaker, coach, and educator specializing in the areas of relationship wellness, empowerment, and LGBTQ faith-based trauma. She is the founder of Pink Love Wellness, LLC, and LGBTQ Faith Matters. A pageant queen, Renair holds the title of Ms. Exquisite Full-Figured USA At-Large 2021. She has a Master of Arts in Religious Education along with a Doctor of Ministry degree. Dr. Amin resides in Queens, New York.

Brendan Y. Boone

The Rev. Brendan Y. Boone (he/him), a native Virginian, has been a member of Metropolitan Community Churches (MCC) for over thirty-five years and has served in several denominational leadership capacities. A graduate of the Hampton Institute and Wesley Theological Seminary, Rev. Boone has served MCCs in Virginia, The District of Columbia, North Carolina, and Florida. He and his wife, Sandra, now reside in Daytona Beach, Florida, with their four-legged child, Maximilian Cooper Boone.

Allen V. Harris

Allen V. Harris (he/him) serves as the Regional Pastor and President of the Christian Church in Ohio. Previously he served as the Regional Minister of the Christian Church Capital Area and a local church pastor in Cleveland, Ohio, New York, New York, and Grapevine, Texas. Allen was ordained in 1991 as an openly gay man and has been a leader in the GLAD Alliance (now AllianceQ) since its inception. He cofounded the Open & Affirming Ministries Program.

Marian Edmonds-Allen

Rev. Marian Edmonds-Allen (she/they) is the executive director of Parity and the director of Blessed by Difference, a project that seeks to promote curious and collaborative bridging across the LGBTQ+ and faith divide. Marian has worked with youth and families in various denominations and settings throughout the country for more than twenty years, focusing on strengths-based interventions and supports to affirm beliefs and faith practices for LGBTQ+ people.

Acknowledgements

The *Introduction* highlights the importance of naming: "To name and to call by name is a powerful, brave, life-giving act." And so with gratitude I name:

The *Colors of Hope* co-creator Alysha Laperche who in my first two months of employment with AllianceQ asked if they could be an intern. Alysha, thank you for your life-giving ministry as an intern and now as a Co-Moderator as well as your friendship.

The contributors to this manifestation of *Colors of Hope:*

Tyler Heston, who also held (and affirmed and enriched) my potential and the potential of this book at the very beginnings.

Sandhya Jha, Nadia Tavera, and Andrew Deeb.

William DeShay C. Jackson who wrote about my favorite color yellow and brought light to my life across the miles.

Renair Amin and Brendan Y. Boone, both of whom added their voices because of the Spirit's real prompting and presence. Brendan is one of my pastors and our stories have come full circle, encompassing change and transformation.

Allen V. Harris who has deep roots with the Alliance, having stretched himself and the church, expanding our understanding and reach.

Marian Edmonds-Allen who is a bridge builder. They just have a way of helping me make a way. I always find encouragement and motivation in Marian.

These contributors to the original *Colors of Hope* podcast series not otherwise listed:

Sophia Jackson, YaNi Davis, Chaim "CJ" Rodriguez, Cameron Van Kooten Laughead, Kyle Miller-Shawnee, Logan Rozos, Michael Marren Jennys, and Chrissy Stonebraker-Martinez.

AllianceQ – the Disciples LGBTQ+ Alliance and its Council Members, current and past. Especially Moderators and friends Luther Young, Robin Knauerhase, and Dan Adolphson.

Bob Shaw, former Council Member, trusted colleague, and committed ally with a lot of wisdom and a few good jokes.

Mark Johnston, who also has deep roots with the Alliance, directing and inspiring much of the Open & Affirming ministry in the Christian Church (Disciples of Christ), and who equipped me to serve as Executive Director + Minister.

Alliance members who donate their resources, time, and many incredible talents to widen the welcome and witness to God's expansive love. There are too many members to name, but Ben Bohren and Jimmy Spear have been cheerleaders—for the work and me.

Disciples Justice Ministries. We are better together, striving to understand and working for intersectional justice. Ally and colleague Brian Frederick-Gray with Disciples Peace Fellowship may not know that his spirit and leadership have been inspirational.

Amber Churchill. I want to be like them (and I think they have some hope in me).

Terri Hord Owens. She is a faithful leader for the Christian Church (Disciples of Christ) and an ally. She mentors me directly and indirectly.

Lee Hull Moses, first a colleague and now a friend, who has supported my family in dark valleys and celebrated bright moments.

I name formative communities, places, and people:

Salvage Garden and its founding leaders Cindy Good and Brian Russell. Dwight Meredith who for some reason believes in me more than anyone else and supports me and my family through life's (changing and complicated) seasons. I want to be as compassionate and generous as Dwight Meredith. Gia Gaster.

First Christian Church Greensboro. Sue Hulighan. Diana Huth. Cliff and Louise Greaves. Beverly Isaacson. Barbara Gillespie. JoAnn Tucker.

Susan Cox, builder and listener. What friend will tattoo a spoon on their body to share in your "tear soup"?

Wake Forest University School of Divinity. Professors and colleagues Jill Crainshaw and Diane Lipsett. Wow. There are no words. Amber Harris who I met at Wake, who understands me in profoundly deep ways and annoyingly calls me to be my best self.

Wartburg College. Ramona Bouzard and Larry Trachte. They published some of my first writing and endorsed *A Knight's Armor.* Jake Sorenson.

Rainbow Trail Lutheran Camp. Trinity Lutheran Church. Pastor Gregg and Kris Davison. "PG" was my childhood pastor, part of my faith formation and call to ministry. The mountaintop experiences were life changing. And all the meals! Kris, thank you for the meals throughout youth ministry and more importantly your kindness and support.

There are also friends and family. Some meaning-makers who sustained my hope or hoped for me when I felt hopeless. Melissa Hosey and Shannon Dalkey. The Proudfits. Jeff Sharpe. James Thomas for reviewing job applications and book manuscripts, providing theological conversation best paired with hard cider, and letting me borrow his truck all the time. Pastor Sebastian Shepherd who knows a bit about love and loss and hoping in color.

My sister-in-law Jarrett Joyce. Mother-in-law Cindi Vernon. Sister-in-law Natalie Loy. My sister Michelle who is strong and resilient and somehow more stubborn than me. She has an annoying positivity that I hope moves her to deep joy. My mother Debra to whom I am indebted—literally and spiritually—and for whom I hope these stories of hope are transformative.

My wife Leah. My children Stephanie, Tommy, Josie, and Orie. You fill every day with color!

Chalice Press and Brad Lyons, thank you for reaching out. Thank you for embodying God's love for every body.

A Note on Language

from

Colors of Hope is a devotional journal *from* LGBTQ+ Christians not a devotional journal (exclusively) *for* LGBTQ+ Christians. It is a resource for every body, for the LGBTQ+ community *and* the wider church.

LGBTQ+

Lesbian, Gay, Bisexual, Transgender, Queer

We use LGBTQ+ for an expansive community represented by a range of initialisms. We acknowledge that language and identity are constantly evolving. Read more about initialisms, definitions, and binaries in the About AllianceQ section.

+

Plus what?

Because our language is limited, because language is bound up in our personal histories and cultural assumptions, language sometimes serves as a barrier instead of bridge to understanding.

+ is an invitation to redefine, further define, and imagine *more*.

It's also a creative representation of the space between and beyond...

Pronouns

Alysha Laperche explains, "Pronouns are used in everyday speech and writing to take the place of people's names. We frequently use pronouns without thinking about them. Often, when speaking of someone in the third person, these pronouns imply a gender. These associations are not always accurate or helpful. Mistaking or assuming peoples' pronouns mistakes their gender and sends a harmful message. Using someone's correct gender pronouns is one of the most basic ways to show your respect for their identity and your love for them."

You may not be familiar with how to use they/them pronouns, but these are the pronouns that Alysha uses. They provide some examples of how to use they/them:

> *"They look amazing in that dress!"*
>
> *"I love how they know it's okay to laugh at themself. They have a great sense of humor."*
>
> *"They are so lucky that Evan is their spouse."*
>
> *"Have you met Alysha yet? That's them over there."*

Practice using pronouns! You'll find more information in Resources.

The New Revised Standard Version (NRSV)

Colors of Hope quotes scripture from the NRSV because it is a familiar, (mostly) accurate translation of our sacred texts. We recognize the many instances of gendered translations for the divine and urge readers to explore a variety of translations. We invite you to consult and consider a range of sources.

Invocation

Shine Through Us

Tyler Heston (he/him)

God who breathes life into each of our bodies,
You speak creativity into chaos,
and all that you make is good.
We are made in your wonder-full image,
bearing your grace, your peace,
your joy, your love.

We are created by you, our creator,
to go out and create:
to make wholeness where things are fragmented,
to sing harmony where things are out of tune,
to fashion peace where there is strife,
and incarnate love where there is hatred.

Forgive us, God, for the places in which we
struggle to embody our faith.
Forgive us for the fragmented identities,
the dissonance between us and you,
the discord we cause with others,
the discrimination we fail to end.

As Jesus confronted people around him
when they twisted your call
empower us to stretch our understanding,
to resist the systems that do harm and dehumanize,
to flip over tables of injustice
that limit the fullness of life
for every body.

Let us see the simplicity
of your all-embracing love.

God who is present with all people:
Lead us and unite us in your Spirit,
She mends together things that are broken.
Send us forward to share your radical love—
a love that discriminates against no person,
a love that celebrates the abundance of ways
that we humans, your creation,
move, love and live.

Hold us together and sustain our hope,
when we are despised for our difference
or when we don't know what to make
of the difference of another.
Shine through us, illuminating our rainbow colors,
so that we, your people,
form a mosaic made in your image,
where beauty, hope, healing, and love
color every corner.

Amen.

An Introduction to *Colors of Hope*

"This is who I am!"

Alysha Laperche (they/them)

What does hope look like in our changing landscape? What color is hope?

Gilbert Baker created the original Pride flag in 1978 to spark courage in the LGBTQ+[1] community, offering a means of proclaiming, "This is who I am!"[2] In a world where discrimination and hatred range from shame and dismissal to physical violence, it takes hope and courage for LGBTQ+ people to be "out," to proclaim, "This is who I am!"

Journalists and historians write that Baker was urged by Harvey Milk, the first openly gay person to be elected to public office in California, to devise a new symbol of pride. The original flag had eight stripes. Pink stood for sexuality, red for life, orange for healing, yellow for sunlight, green for nature, turquoise for magic or art, blue for harmony or serenity, and purple for spirit. What theme would you assign to each color?

How can we individually and collectively hope in color?

Hope is an act of resistance, challenging and dismantling systemic injustices that rob people of wholeness and wellness—that deprive us of hope. It resists the depression and despair that swirl within us and around us. To hope is to imagine and shape a new reality: a brighter

---

[1]The initialism for "Lesbian, Gay, Bisexual, Transgender, and Queer." Sometimes denoted with different or additional letters.

[2]"How Did the Rainbow Flag Become a Symbol of LGBTQ Pride?" *Encyclopedia Britannica*, accessed September 25, 2021, https://www.britannica.com/story/how-did-the-rainbow-flag-become-a-symbol-of-lgbt-pride.

future, a more just and inclusive world. The hope of our ancestors in the LGBTQ+ community carries us into the present moment.

If it weren't for those who came before us—their struggles, their witness, their hope—we would not be where we are today. In the United States, we have equal marriage rights, an out gay man ran for president, and there are Pride parades on the streets of some of the most unexpected towns. But we are far from fulfilling our hopes for justice and equity. Still, we must recognize that we are living in the hope of those who came before us. It is now our turn to hope in color, imagining and shaping that just future where the expansive love of God is embodied in every aspect of life.

You might be *wondering* about these LGBTQ+ ancestors. Well...

Marsha P. Johnson *resisted* the brutality of the police at Stonewall[3] and became a Queer icon.

Sylvia Rivera, also involved in the riots at Stonewall, *embodied* the LGBTQ+ community's concept of "chosen family" in her bond with Marsha P. Johnson, saying that Johnson was "like a mother."[4] And Rivera sought to establish safe spaces for queer homeless youth.

Gilbert Baker *created* a symbol to represent the great expanse of identities and individuals in the LGBTQ+ community and utilized art for activism.

A Disciples of Christ church in Lynchburg, Virginia, *stretched* that Pride flag across its church building, and I drove by it every day on my way to and from an internship my junior year of college at Liberty University. The public display of the Pride flag *stretched* my view of the church, prompting me to realize *I wasn't alone.*

I *shared* my story of self-awareness and affirmation with the pastor of that congregation years later. The minister wrote, "That's what the flag symbolizes to us: *hope.* We *hoped* the Pride flag would remind people that they are never alone."

Wonder. Resist. Embody. Create. Stretch. Share. Hope.

---

[3]The Stonewall riots in New York City on June 28, 1969, are considered the beginning of the LGBTQ+ rights movement.

[4]"Sylvia Rivera," *National Women's History Museum*, accessed September 25, 2021, https://www.womenshistory.org/education-resources/biographies/sylvia-rivera.

These are the invitations extended to you. You'll find journal prompts for each of these calls to action for each color + theme of the Pride flag.

Colors of Hope was born in the spring of 2020 during my tenure as an intern with AllianceQ – the Disciples LGBTQ+ Alliance, in the heat of the COVID-19 pandemic. This is who I am:

My name is *Alysha* which means "noble one." I am part of the Christian Church (Disciples of Christ) which calls itself a movement for wholeness in a fragmented world. And I serve with AllianceQ. The Alliance strives to foster intentional relationships.

Names have meaning. What we call something or someone implicitly or explicitly illustrates our perceptions and values about the object, topic, or person. In that way, the names that we give and the names that we use are forms of power in our everyday conversations, just as refraining from naming something or someone is a powerful choice and expression.

One ministry concentration for the Alliance is cultivating and supporting Open & Affirming Ministries. Open & Affirming? "O&A?" What does that mean? Part of its interpretation is contextual. Especially as Disciples, we exist within our respective locations, and our theological beliefs frame the meaning and implications of "O&A." Even so, beyond the designation as an Open & Affirming Ministry there is a deep call to embody the teachings of Jesus. The question for congregations and organizations is: "What are we doing to actively embody an expansive welcome and affirmation for all people, reflective of the all-encompassing love of God?"

Designation as an O&A ministry is not the powerful, world-changing thing in and of itself. It is the hope-filled courage to specifically name and give witness to what open & affirming ministry looks like in one's own context. A crucial part of the Open & Affirming process is developing a Welcome Statement. Born out of intentional conversations in the faith community, these statements specifically name the communities—and therefore, the peoples—with whom the congregation or organization wants to show hospitality, welcome, and affirmation.

AllianceQ has examples of statements. An Open & Affirming or Welcome Statement is a way of sharing the heart and identity of the congregation or organization. It reflects the present reality as well as the imagined vision for the future as we all move toward wholeness, as we ever-unfold, becoming more reflective of God's expansive love through our named and practiced inclusion.

Folks may wonder: What is so important about taking the time to specifically *name* all of that? My church already welcomes everyone! Why do we need to write a statement? Why do we need to proclaim that we are an Open & Affirming Ministry?

Because Jesus models for us the practice of intentionality. Because Jesus calls people by their names. Jesus calls Mary by her name after the resurrection when, in her grief, she is searching for meaning and truth during a confusing time (John 20). Jesus calls Lazarus by name into regeneration and life (John 11).

To name and to call by name is a powerful, brave, life-giving act. Naming is an embodiment of the personal God we worship, the God who Jesus taught us so much about.

There is a difference for me between hearing, "everyone is welcome here" and hearing, "you, Alysha, are welcome here." I invite us to consider who our ministries and organizations are naming and thereby intentionally welcoming. Who are we assuming will know they are welcome and will find belonging? Who is missing from the table?

Colors of Hope (COH) names LGBTQ+ Christians. COH offers a sense of belonging for LGBTQ+ people of faith. There is a connection with the faith journeys of LGBTQ+ people and their experiences with scripture that are liberating, meaningful, and hopeful. COH uses LGBTQ+ for an expansive community represented by a range of initialisms. We acknowledge that language and identity are constantly evolving.

What began as a series of podcasts has evolved to serve as a source of empowerment for LGBTQ+ Christians and allies. Many LGBTQ+ Christians have been told that we are not fit to teach, preach, or speak in a faith context because of who we are and how we love. Just as a rainbow stretches across an expanse of the sky, *Colors of Hope* stretches an expanse of identities, locations, ages, abilities, genders, and more.

The podcasts feature reflections from queer faith leaders that explore a lectionary text alongside a color and theme from Gilbert Baker's

Pride flag. This is queer: Contributors were asked to stretch and create a reflection that integrated seemingly disparate components. Each series launched eight weeks before Pride, the month of June, with one color + theme highlighted each week. The ninth reflection on The Rainbow served as a bridge to Pride month.

Rainbows are plastered everywhere during Pride month. We all know that when Pride month concludes individual and corporate social media profiles pivot from all-rainbows-all-the-time to whatever they looked like on May 31. Pride—and the fierce urgency for hope—must stretch beyond a single month, filling every single day and every single space with color.

This devotional journal is an adaptation of the podcast series with expanded content and unique journal prompts. *Colors of Hope* is a resource for every body, for the LGBTQ+ community *and* the wider church, lifting up the call to embody our faith. For our allies, family members, and those who want to learn more, the devotions and journal prompts provide opportunities to engage scripture and explore worldviews outside of or beyond one's own context.

According to Baker, the Pride flag expresses joy, beauty, and power. There's power in proclamation: "This is who I am!" *This is who we are!* And there's power in hope. Hope as an act of resistance. Hope as an embodiment of our faith.

"Hoping in color" brings the joy, beauty, and power of the rainbow to life.

Here's to hoping in color.

Pink + Sex

There's a ballroom in heaven, and there's room for you on the dance floor

Sandhya Jha (she/they)

Now the whole group of those who believed were of one heart and soul, and no one claimed private ownership of any possessions, but everything they owned was held in common. With great power the apostles gave their testimony to the resurrection of the Lord Jesus, and great grace was upon them all. There was not a needy person among them, for as many as owned lands or houses sold them and brought the proceeds of what was sold. They laid it at the apostles' feet, and it was distributed to each as any had need. (Acts 4:32–35)

Until this project, I had never thought too deeply about the LGBTQ+ flag as a historic resource. I also didn't realize pink was one of the colors in the flag. And when I found out the pink stripe represented sexuality, and also that it would be part of a devotional, I felt a little daunted.

However, as I began to dig into that history, I found myself captivated by Gilbert Baker's story of how this flag came to be the symbol for the LGBTQ+ movement. Visiting the Winterland Ballroom in the 1970s, a gay dance club in San Francisco, Baker said:

> Everyone was there. North Beach beatniks and barrio zoots, the bored bikers in black leather, teenagers in the back row kissing. There were long-haired, lithe girls in belly-dance get-ups; pink-haired punks safety-pinned together; hippie suburbanites; movie stars so beautiful they left you dumbstruck; muscle gay boys with perfect mustaches; butch

dykes in blue jeans; and fairies of all genders in thrift-store dresses. We rode the mirrored ball on glittering LSD and love power. Dance fused us, magical and cleansing. We were all in a swirl of color and light. It was like a rainbow.[5]

And so the rainbow flag was conceived, at a dance club in the Castro.

Gilbert Baker's flag has evolved a lot over the years. A version that moved me deeply a few years ago was one that added a black and a brown stripe and my favorite one of today includes on the side a chevron of black and brown (for cross-racial solidarity) and pink, white, and blue (to explicitly represent the trans community).

Additionally, a few colors dropped out, one of which is the bright hot pink stripe that Gilbert Baker chose to represent sexuality.

There's an old joke about the church's stance on sex that says: "Sex is dirty; save it for someone you love."

And the passage we ground ourselves in seems on its face to have nothing to do with sex.

It might feel like a stretch to connect an erased stripe of sexuality with an iconic passage about Christian community...but how much of a stretch is it, really?

That story of the earliest church is almost magical: "No one claimed private ownership of any possessions, but everything they owned was held in common...There was not a needy person among them for as many as owned lands or houses sold them and brought the proceeds of what was sold." It makes sense that the early church would have functioned in such inclusive ways so early on. The folks at the center of the church in the book of Acts had real life encounters with Jesus and the Holy Spirit. I imagine that brush with the sacred would have made creating heaven on earth almost urgent.

There is something profound about this passage, something that grounds me in what I want the church to be, what I long for in the church. Something that, despite disappointments with our inability to recreate it, I keep aspiring to an experience of real, absolute joy; joy like those disciples knew having encountered the risen Christ.

---

[5]David Lewis, "The Rainbow Warrior," *San Francisco Magazine,* June 14, 2019. https://sanfran.com/the-rainbow-warrior.

I don't often find a sustained version of it. But I do encounter glimpses of it.

This passage from the book of Acts is in many ways why I wanted to be a minister in the first place: to be part of a community like this.

And it might be hard to see what that has to do with sexuality, but bear with me.

In the spring of 2021, I was accepted into an artists' residency to research any subject I wanted to as a queer artist of color. I chose to delve into the lives of South Asian immigrant LGBTQQIA[6] ancestors. My hope was that what I learned could offer a source of encouragement and inspiration to those of us navigating our experiences today.

I wanted to connect with ancestors. The ancestors whispered a word that a lot of the research was going to be painful because most of the records we have of South Asian immigrant ancestors in the US are criminal records from times they were prosecuted for pursuing their desires. And so the ancestors told me they wanted me to focus on joy and resilience and power. I'm grateful they did because I needed those glimpses of joy amidst so much heartbreak.

I share with you a documentary I came across in my research, called *Khush*. "Khush" is a word that in Hindi or Urdu translates to happiness or really to ecstatic pleasure. And it's a word that in the seventies and eighties the underground LGBTQ+ movement in India claimed as their self-defining terminology—men and women alike and people across the gender spectrum. Khush.

In the documentary, members of the queer community were asked, "What is good about being khush?" I remember one man in the documentary saying two things: the desire and the siblinghood.

The desire and the siblinghood.

Now what strikes me as profound is this: the same longing, the same passion, the same seeking joy that my ancestors wanted for me is what brought them joy about identifying as queer. The desire and the siblinghood.

---

[6]Lesbian, Gay, Bisexual, Transgender, Queer, Questioning, Intersex, and Allies

It's the same experience I have as I dream of what church could be. Those longings are not so different.

The other thing I find important is the folks in the Winterland Ballroom experienced, whether it was in all of their lives or just for the hours they were in that space, a freedom in being who they were, without having to hide any part of their true selves. Like the urgency the early church felt in creating heaven on earth because of their brush with the sacred, there is a brush with the sacred that creates the same sense of urgency for building heaven on earth within the queer community I am part of. And to us, heaven on earth means everyone's needs being met, everyone's gifts being honored, and people not having to hide who they are to be safe...just like in the early church.

I think something we forget about the early church is that—while they were persecuted, while they were countercultural, while they were under threat—they were willing to risk all of that for the freedom to finally be the community they had always wanted to be. A longing got fulfilled.

It got fulfilled in community.

Something I didn't mention about Gilbert Baker's flag is that he was seeking to replace the omnipresent pink triangle with something more life-giving and joyful. It was profoundly countercultural for the LGBTQ+ community to reclaim that pink triangle, the symbol the Nazis had used to mark "known homosexuals" in concentration camps. Reclaiming the pink triangle was about saying that we in the queer community refused to let the world force us to hide who we were or be ashamed of who we were; yet that pink triangle was also a reminder that we had been and still were and still are persecuted, marginalized, oppressed.

The early church and the early LGBTQ+ rights movement both knew persecution. And they both knew they had a fundamental right to joy and community.

So I love that while Baker eschewed the triangle for something more resplendent, he kept the pink and connected it to the thing we are supposed to be ashamed of—our desire.

Gilbert Baker's pink stripe representing sexuality didn't disappear because it was too controversial but for a much more practical reason.

When the demand for rainbow flags spiked after the murder of Harvey Milk, hot pink was too expensive and too rare a fabric to find, costing us one of our stripes. But I hope we don't forget what it has to offer us as Christians committed to queer liberation, to liberation for all.

When Gilbert Baker included sex as part of the proclamation of what LGBTQ+ folks could reclaim as a source of pride, he was inviting us to reclaim the very thing that we were shamed for wanting. It was the thing that we were shamed for pursuing.

By proclaiming sexuality boldly and unapologetically, Gilbert Baker was offering us freedom. Not freedom to do whatever we wanted whenever we wanted no matter what with no consequences, but freedom to be part of a community that was unapologetic about its desire and about its willingness to show up for each other.

I don't think that Gilbert Baker's experience of the Winterland Ballroom in San Francisco with the North Beach beatniks and the hippies, suburbanites, and the butch dykes in blue jeans—and I include that one again because I resonate with it—was all that different from the persecuted and joyous, countercultural and thriving community in the book of Acts.

I founded a nonprofit called the Oakland Peace Center. At our very founding, at the very launch of the Oakland Peace Center, we had a panel of leaders of color from the community across several generations who were giving us advice on how to not burn out in the midst of the work of Justice.

One of those people was the Reverend Phil Lawson, a key leader in the nonviolent resistance movement you might know as the civil rights movement, which its leaders actually called the US Freedom Movement. Reverend Phil said to our group, "I need you to remember: the opposite of slavery isn't freedom. The opposite of slavery is community."

I am really proud to be representing one of the hardest-to-theologize colors in the rainbow flag.

I'm proud because, in proclaiming my desire, I'm proclaiming my community.

In proclaiming my desire, I'm proclaiming my freedom.

In proclaiming my desire, I'm claiming the church in a whole new way.

And I hope you'll join me in that reclamation.

Wonder

Imagine that dance floor at the Winterland Ballroom as heaven. Who do you see on the dance floor? Who are they dancing with? Who's DJing? What music is playing?

Resist

Imagine those South Asian gay immigrants from 100 years ago; picture their mug shots or imagine them walking the yard at Folsom Prison.

What is Jesus calling you to do that makes a better world for their descendants? (Their biological, spiritual, or justice movement descendants.)

Embody

What does desire feel like for you, physically? Do different types of desire feel different?

What longings do you hold? What longings do you have for the church?

What are your feelings telling you about what you might be called to do?

Create

What does it look like to build a community that offers an alternative to persecution and mistreatment? Who is involved in shaping it? Picture your own role in creating that type of community, and who is building it with you.

Where do you experience siblinghood? How was that created? If you lack siblinghood, how will you begin to create it?

Hope

The author talked about proclaiming their desire as a way of celebrating and honoring their community. What desires do you want to proclaim, and how will they connect you to the Holy Spirit?

What proclamations might help you experience freedom?

Stretch

What would it look like to engage in meaningful conversation with your faith community about sexuality as part of our human and divine experience? Where would that start? Where might it lead? Who could journey with you?

Share

If you were to share with someone the story of the pink stripe in the Pride flag, what would you want them to know? What else might it allow you to discuss?

Begin the conversation.

Red + Life

Una Fuente de Esperanza

Nadia Tavera (she/they)

*See what love the Father has given us, that we should be called
children of God; and that is what we are. The reason the world
does not know us is that it did not know him. Beloved, we are
God's children now; what we will be has not yet been revealed.
What we do know is this: when he is revealed, we will be like
him, for we will see him as he is. And all who have this hope in
him purify themselves, just as he is pure. Everyone who commits
sin is guilty of lawlessness; sin is lawlessness. You know that he
was revealed to take away sins, and in him there is no sin. No
one who abides in him sins; no one who sins has either seen him
or known him. Little children, let no one deceive you. Everyone
who does what is right is righteous, just as he is righteous. (1
John 3:1–7)*

Red has a range of symbolic meanings. I've been told that our ancestors
saw red as the color of fire and blood, as energy flowing from the heart.
The heart is more than a vital organ or romantic symbol. Rather, it
refers to an intangible composition of our soul that is the seat of life,
where the deepest feelings of our being are housed. In the depths of
your being, know that *you are a child of God.*

The 1 John scripture—and many others—affirm that you
and I are God's beloved children. The word "children" in the original
Greek is τέκνα (tekna). The verb ἐσμέν (esmen) follows and is used in
present active indicative form, which means "we are!" The affirmation
that we are children of God appears twice in the same paragraph.
We are God's children. I needed to hear this twice. I needed to hear

it over and over. And over. It took numerous affirmations to embrace the fullness of my identity. *I am a child of God.*

Like Gilbert Baker's proclamation, "This is who I am!" I proclaim, "We are children of God!"

I understand the Divine to be a God of life and a God of love.

But for many years I couldn't accept that God loved me because I am gay. They were the worst years of my life—if it could be called life. I could not reconcile my faith and sexual orientation. Feeling rejected by God caused deep wounds in my being.

In my early years, I found myself in non-affirming spaces where homosexuality was seen as evil. I was a teenager who loved God and enjoyed attending church every Sunday. Nobody knew I was gay because homosexuals were not recognized as children of God by my faith community.

"...The reason the world does not know us is that it did not know him... what we will be has not yet been revealed..."

My mom took me to church since I was four years old. She believed in submission. She held strong beliefs about gender roles. I struggled with why I was not allowed to do the same things as my brother Edgar, like riding a bike or going out to play with friends. I had to stay at home, helping my mom with chores. I found refuge in my studies to avoid the imposition of "female" roles. I stayed in the closet; I pretended to be straight to be accepted by my parents.

I remember I prayed fervently for a change. I thought God wanted me to be straight. I prayed and fasted, and nothing happened. I still felt physical attraction to other women. I was twelve years old when I started struggling with something that I was unable to change. I wanted to please God, but I could not be called their child according to the norm. I was afraid of being expelled from my faith community, so I pretended to be what I was not.

Over the years I developed a sense of self-loathing that became ingrained in my heart, in my spirit. I remember that every time my gay identity flared up, a feeling of guilt came over me.

For a long time, I repressed my sexual orientation and gender identity. I decided not to come out to please my family and eventually to keep a job. Deep down, I knew I was still gay. My conscience condemned me, and the self-loathing increased. I came into adulthood as an introvert with low self-esteem. Not being recognized as a child of God led to internalized homophobia, anxiety, and depression.

My life was dominated by the struggle of wanting to please God and be myself. The negative voices that shouted I was not a beloved child of God were the only voices I heard.

I could no longer pretend to be straight, so I stopped attending church and began to explore my sexual orientation. I met LGBTQ+ groups that supported me, enabling me to "come out." I was afraid of being despised by my family and I was afraid of losing my job, so I did not come out completely. I revealed only parts of myself to certain parts of my community.

"...The reason the world does not know us is that it did not know him... what we will be has not yet been revealed. What we do know is this: when he is revealed, we will be like him, for we will see him as he is."

I could be myself with other queer folks, but I pretended to be someone else in non-affirming spaces.

Finally, years later, I found La Comunidad Cristiana de Esperanza (The Christian Community of Hope), the first open and affirming church in Mexico City. The services were like the church where I grew up, but the leadership was different. A cisgender[7] gay man preached that gay folks were beloved children of God. Sermons focused on grace instead of law. Pastor Ricardo often said, "You don't have to do anything or stop doing something to be loved by God." What a revelation!

I didn't yet embrace it fully...

At that time, I was twenty-six years old. The negative voices echoed in my mind. I still heard condemnation. But I was beginning to glimpse acceptance and love. It was hard for me to believe that I was a beloved child of God, but I decided to explore what the preacher affirmed, and I continued to attend the church. It took me several months to accept that God affirms me as I am and calls me their child. I had to release the oppressive biblical interpretations and read scripture with new lenses, with the lenses of God's love. It was

---

[7]Cisgender: someone whose gender identity corresponds with the sex the person was assigned at birth.

a process. It still is a process! The expansive love of God continues to be revealed to me.

When I think about the complex mental and spiritual process I journeyed through, my experience as a computer programmer comes to mind. For more than ten years, I coded algorithms for the financial industry, and computer programming informs me that my mind works like a machine that processes ideas based on input. For those unfamiliar with programming languages, coding an algorithm is writing a series of instructions that the computer can understand to process information automatically. Regardless of the amount or diversity of data, the computer will always process the information in the same way.

Those who have experience in coding know that even the best programmer may code an algorithm incorrectly and the outcome will be inaccurate. See where I'm going here? Something similar happened to me when I was in non-affirming spaces. My mind was coded with oppressive social norms and biblical interpretations. Since the human mind is more complex than computers, the negative words affected my brain, my soul, my whole being.

I wonder, what have you learned and from whom did you learn? What have you learned about scripture? About gender and sexuality? About race and class? About… And what are your sources?

"Little children, let no one deceive you…"

During my time at La Comunidad Cristiana de Esperanza, my mind processed a range of new input. I did exhaustive exegetical studies of the Bible. And the people around me affirmed me as a child of God beloved by God. The good news of God's love for all reprogrammed my brain. My understanding of God and self and community were transformed. Finally, I was able to receive the great love of the Father as a gay woman. God restored my mind and started healing my soul. It was a new beginning that allowed me to live more fully.

I can testify that the love of God set me free from shame and guilt. Recognizing that I am a child of God encourages me to share my experience with other folks looking to live the life that God has prepared for them. It requires a lot of courage, self-confidence, and trust in God.

Three years ago, I moved to San Francisco, California, to attend seminary. Living far away from family, I found the courage I needed to embody my gender identity. I altered my feminine look. I adopted the masculine identity that I always longed for. I was angry with myself for having repressed my gender identity for so many years. And I stopped talking to my parents because they weren't willing to affirm me. My family and I were very close until I came out.

After one year of distancing, the reconciliation between me and my parents happened. I texted my mother saying that I couldn't keep pretending and her support was very important to me. She took three days before responding. She told me it was hard for her to accept who I am, but she loves me because I'm her daughter. She also expressed that she and my dad have always been proud of me. Love won. And every day my parents and I learn how to express the love we feel for each other.

"...when God is revealed, we will be like him, for we will see him as he is. And all who have this hope in God purify themselves, just as God is pure."

Every day I remind myself that I'm a beloved child of God. God calls me Her beloved child!

I repeat this mantra I learned from a spiritual coach: "I accept myself as I am and forgive myself for all the time that I couldn't bear to be me." The daily exercise sparks courage. It strengthens my self-confidence and deepens my trust in God.

Finally, I want to share that my theology about salvation and sin changed when I embraced God's grace that came with their love. I believe that salvation is here and now and has to do with bringing someone from a state of oppression to a state of liberation. Being in community is key to dismantling oppressive systems. Spending time with others to listen to them is vitally important. Our actions are important. We cannot tell somebody that God loves them apart from demonstrating our love for one another.

For those facing oppression because of their sexual orientation and/or gender identity, I pray that my testimony may be a source of hope—una fuente de esperanza—and that all people may be affirmed in God's expansive, life-giving love.

"See what love the Father has given us."

One more reference to Greek. The word translated as "see" has its root in the Greek verb εἴδω (eído) that means recognize and understand. Translations use the following words: See. Behold. Know. Consider. Cherish.

It is a source of hope to "consider the kind of extravagant love the Parent has lavished on us—He calls us children of God! It's true; we are Her beloved children."[8]

Cherish this love.

---

[8]Author's adaptation of 1 John 3:1 from *The Voice*. Author varies gendered pronouns for God.

Wonder

Explore the ways you formed your beliefs. What have you learned about scripture? About gender and sexuality? About race and class? About... And what are your sources?

Resist

Has a person or group said you are not a beloved child of God? Or have you felt unlovable? How do you resist those messages and reprogram your mind?

Embody

Gilbert Baker paired the color red with life. The author refers to red as the color of fire and blood, as energy flowing from the heart. What do you associate with the color red?

How does the color feel? Hot, passionate, energizing, scary?

Create

What "exercise" can spark courage? Strengthen your self-confidence? Deepen your trust in God?

Write your own mantra and/or find affirmations to repeat (to yourself and to share with others).

Hope

The author described their experience at La Comunidad Cristiana de Esperanza (The Christian Community of Hope)—where they literally found hope. In what community or communities have you found hope?

If you long for such community, how will you seek to be in community?

Stretch

In their writing the author uses a range of pronouns for God. Is it a stretch for you to do this?

What aspects of God can be revealed to us by reimagining gendered imagery in the Bible?

Colors of Hope uses the *New Revised Standard Version.* Consider adapting the gendered imagery as you continue this journey.

How do gendered roles in the home and in society limit us? How do you (or how will you) challenge stereotypes and gender roles?

Share

The author refers to her story as a testimony and says, "I pray that my testimony may be a source of hope—una fuente de esperanza..." Write about something from your faith journey that could be a source of hope for someone else.

Consider sharing your story.

Orange + Healing

Still Here

Andrew Deeb (he/him)

Blessed be the God and Father of our Lord Jesus Christ! By his great mercy he has given us a new birth into a living hope through the resurrection of Jesus Christ from the dead, and into an inheritance that is imperishable, undefiled, and unfading, kept in heaven for you, who are being protected by the power of God through faith for a salvation ready to be revealed in the last time. In this you rejoice, even if now for a little while you have had to suffer various trials, so that the genuineness of your faith—being more precious than gold that, though perishable, is tested by fire—may be found to result in praise and glory and honor when Jesus Christ is revealed. Although you have not seen him, you love him; and even though you do not see him now, you believe in him and rejoice with an indescribable and glorious joy, for you are receiving the outcome of your faith, the salvation of your souls. (1 Peter 1:3–9)

The orange stripe in the Pride flag symbolizes healing. Orange is a bold and vibrant color that when swirled with red and yellow gives us fire and heat. Blended with blues and pinks, orange is also the color of sunsets. Orange is gently dominant among autumn's trees. There is tension between these swatches of color as the bold energy of fire contrasts with the calm and peace in a sunset. The heat of summer contrasts with the coolness of fall. A tension exists in healing, too. Healing is a process. What was and what will be forges resolution, regeneration, repair, and restoration.

The 1 Peter passage promises healing and evokes faith in the ensuing process. The scripture celebrates a healing already made manifest,

"...by his great mercy he has given us a new birth into a living hope through the resurrection of Jesus Christ..." And the scripture affirms a healing that will manifest, "...to be revealed in the last time..." It is the promise of our salvation, which I understand to be the restoration of creation and perfect harmony with God. Salvation is wellness and wholeness: for individuals, communities, and the world. God's promise, symbolized in the fullness of the rainbow, will never change.

I like the language used in the New Living Translation (NLT):

> "...Now we live with great expectation, and we have a priceless inheritance—an inheritance that is kept in heaven for you, pure and undefiled, beyond the reach of change and decay. And through your faith, God is protecting you..." (1 Peter 1:3–5)

Our "priceless inheritance," our healing and wholeness, the text suggests, is the outcome of our faith. What is faith though? Growing up in a conservative tradition in the Midwest, I was taught that having faith meant inviting Jesus into your heart, going to church, reading the Bible. While there is nothing necessarily wrong with such things, they do not capture the fullness of faith as I understand it. Faith is more than our beliefs; faith is our beliefs enacted. To me, faith is existing in and refusing to back down from spaces of tension. It is declaring life in the face of death, love in the face of apathy. Sometimes living in faith, living out our faith, is choosing to put one foot in front of the other, persevering when surrounded by uncertainty and chaos. To heal, we navigate the tensions and move forward.

As we move forward, we will inevitably face trials and suffering. Trials and suffering shape us. But God does not cause us to suffer to make us stronger. Suffering is the nature of living in a broken world. I long for—and work for—the restoration of creation.

"There is a wonderful joy ahead..." (1 Peter 1:6 NLT)

The text offers the example of fire burning away impurities in gold. I think of welding. Metal heats to create a bond. A good weld is strong. It won't break even under the most immense strain. As with welding, our faith passes through the fire, melts down, and fuses together with something new, forging something stronger. The result is a product new and old. This is healing. Our wounded selves never return to who we were before; rather, we move forward empowered by all the experiences.

Healing. Not a return but resolution, regeneration, repair, and restoration.

When I came out as trans, I felt the heat and my faith was tested by orange-red flames that manifested through discrimination and harassment. My connections with community were extinguished. I lost friends and family members. I faced hate and hurt where I was attending school and there came a point that I had to transfer. I was ousted by my church, the family I thought knew me and accepted me. I was barred from communion within the entire denomination.

Those who inflicted these wounds used God's love as justification for rejecting and mistreating me. They told me that who I am is fundamentally wrong, that I would be an agent of the devil if I decided to "live in sin." One person told me that God would rather have me dead than be trans. I was thrown into a fire with no idea what would burn up and what, if anything, would come out reforged.

I eventually emerged, alive but undeniably changed. I encountered a living, loving God who wanted me to live and live in the fullness of my identity. My previous conceptions of God's judgement and sin were found lacking and melted away. Even though some of the people closest to me rejected me and abandoned me, others rose to support me. A family from my former church took me in and made sure I knew I had a place. My relationship with my parents eventually began to mend. God showed up in unexpected ways to let me know I was loved, to stress that I was not alone, to push me forward.

One encounter with God sticks with me, reminding me who God is even when I feel lost. I wandered into a random worship service somewhere on campus. I was in a wounded state, suffering deeply, reeling from the loss of relationships that were so important to me. And I wasn't sure if God, too, had abandoned me. I wondered if God hated me. I didn't know why I wandered into the worship, but I felt restless and needed to be anywhere but my apartment. I sat in the back thinking I didn't belong there.

I can't worship God anymore; God is not for people like me.

As my thoughts spiraled, a girl who had been in a cluster of people worshipping at the front came and sat next to me. After a slightly awkward silence, she turned and said, "I know we've never met and this might be weird, but I felt like God wanted me to come tell you how much He loves you and how important you are to Him. Is it alright if me and a couple friends pray over you?"

Complete strangers started praying for me, telling me I was God's beloved son—beloved son! That was a big deal at that point in my life. These strangers asked God to be tangibly present with me in whatever I was going through. I never encountered those students again, but their words stuck with me. Their prayer stuck with me; the prayer awakened in me a profound awareness of God's presence.

And today I sense God tangibly present with me. Each breath of mine is an invocation of the name of God. I see God's artistry in every sunset. I feel the breath of God in the wind blowing through the trees. I see a unique representation of the face of God in every person. I feel the movement and energy of the Spirit in every song. I experience the companionship of Christ in sharing a meal with my friends. These experiences and others like them helped reshape my understanding of God's love, a love more vast and more beautiful than I could have imagined.

Even though I have experienced much healing, I know there is much more to come, more to be revealed. The process of disentangling death-dealing theologies is continual. Healing is not a moment, but a life-long process. God is always with us, though, calling us forward and guiding us through the fire. And there are strangers who will pray for us along the way. There are stunning sunsets at the end of difficult and glorious days.

Sometimes it seems impossible to see through the flames, but because we have faith, because we hope—in color!—we persist. Though we cannot always see God, though it may feel like we don't know who God is or who we are anymore, we press forward. We wander into random worship services...

The church has too frequently modeled for us who God is not. Keep moving. There are faith communities that embody God's inclusive love. Even when told by religious institutions that God does not accept who we are, the way we love, or the people we love, we press forward. Even when we are told that our faith cannot be genuine, we make way. For ourselves and others. Despite everything we have gone through, here we are. Here we are. Our faith must be genuine. We are still here.

And like the writer of 1 Peter, we have a strange but glorious, inexpressible joy. We have joy because we know that healing has already happened, and healing is on the way. We are simultaneously wounded and healed. Joy is wrapped up in grief. Good grief?

Child of God, know that you are the person God created you to be and you were called for such a time as this. In times of death, uncertainty, and pain, you are a beacon of life, love, and healing. Know that even though you may not always feel it, your faith is strong. This faith is an inheritance, from our ancestors and all the saints who have gone before us. The faith of those around you will also sustain you. The fact that you are here, after all you have been through, is testament to the strength of your faith and the life-giving hope of others.

Take heart. Remember that God does not cause suffering for the sake of healing it nor for character development. God does not allow injustice but grieves with us as we work for justice. God does not test us to make sure we really love Them. If we lean on Him in our times of suffering, we come to see that God is right where She promised She would be. God is with us.

Through fires. Sunsets. Hot summers and cool autumn seasons.

Into healing and wholeness. For me. For you. Our communities. Our world.

Wonder

In what ways do you desire healing? What tensions do you experience in the healing process?

Resist

What harmful theologies do you encounter and/or still wrestle with? What are some meaningful ways that you can resist them?

Embody

Describe experiences of healing. Include each of the body's senses. What does healing feel like? Taste like? Sound like?

Create

The author described healing as a process: resolution, regeneration, repair, and restoration. What needs immediate resolution and how can you begin that process?

Regarding material objects, can you repair or restore something? (Not skilled in that way? Seek someone to help you with the process.)

Hope

When "going through the fire," how do you live with "glorious, inexpressible joy"?

What is your vision of a healed world? Describe and/or illustrate healing and wholeness.

Stretch

Is there any part of your belief system, your faith, that might be reforged?

Is there a connection with a person or community you hope to reforge? How will you pursue this?

Share

How will you use your experiences of healing to contribute to the healing of your community and/or the world around you?

Relish someone's indescribable joy and pass it on—the story or the joy or both!

Yellow + Sunlight

Who the Sun Sets Free

William DeShay C. Jackson (they/them)

I am the true vine, and my Father is the vinegrower. He removes every branch in me that bears no fruit. Every branch that bears fruit he prunes to make it bear more fruit. You have already been cleansed by the word that I have spoken to you. Abide in me as I abide in you. Just as the branch cannot bear fruit by itself unless it abides in the vine, neither can you unless you abide in me. I am the vine, you are the branches. Those who abide in me and I in them bear much fruit, because apart from me you can do nothing. (John 15:1–5)

As the Earth rotates to start a new day, it is greeted by the Sun, who bathes the Earth in a warm glow of light and heat. Earth's sky becomes saturated with a tapestry of yellow, orange, and red, cascading from one hemisphere to the next, illuminating everything in its path. Responding to the light of day, creation interacts passively and actively, all under one sun. The Sun, whose energy gives life to all creation, reminds us that we share an abundant resource. Let us link sunlight with the True Vine found in John 15 and explore our connectedness.

My knowledge of trees is limited. I've never planted or pruned a tree. But I do know trees require water, soil, *and sunlight*. And I read that all the parts of a tree, its roots, trunk, branches, and leaves, all the parts play a part in helping the tree use the water, soil, and sunlight.

The John 15 scripture served as the guiding text for the 2019 General Assembly, the biennial gathering of the Christian Church (Disciples of Christ). With the theme "Abide in Me," we were invited to focus on what it means to "abide in God" and "abide in community."

To abide in God suggests a participatory, covenantal relationship. Creator and created. To abide in community, we work together to flourish. Like the parts of a tree. If my branches are sapped, if your branches are unsupported, they will weaken or break, all losing a shared energy. If our branches become entangled, we risk choking ourselves and others. And so we nurture and prune every branch.

No two trees grow to be the same; no two humans are the same, regardless of similar contextual components. Same forest or same family. Our differences need not be daggers for attack but invitations to glimpse our diverse and expansive God. Why not enjoy the fruit each of us brings to the table?

I served as the vice president for the Brite Black Seminarians student group at Brite Divinity. During my tenure I served with two completely different boards. Our work together as an executive board stretched past the meeting space as we spent time fellowshipping around the dinner table, exercising at the gym, and clowning around in Weatherly Hall. Even though I grew up in a historically and predominantly Black Disciples of Christ congregation, those serving on the executive board gave me a glimpse of the array of gifts and personalities that exist amongst melanated, sun-kissed persons. Everyone brought something different to the table. And I was free to exist as my authentic self without apology.

To be Black, nonbinary, and queer is a gift from God, but an unresolved issue to people who project their ignorance or fears onto me. My experience as a nonbinary person and minister has been both an exciting journey of exploration and a painful realization that my identity is considered invalid by some. And sometimes the rationale is linked with grammar!

Growing up in rural northeast Missouri meant that my education in the public school system involved interactions with a sea of persons that did not look like me; nor did we share the same socioeconomic background or access to resources. My blackness was the object of harmful jokes, peers repeating phrases they heard from parents or comedians. My blackness was a target for aggressive looks and near physical altercations. I knew I was Black, but I didn't know that I was allowed to be Black. I didn't know that my blackness was whole enough in certain spaces.

When I came out as queer another part of my community rejected me. Some pretended I was a stranger when we crossed paths in the grocery store. These were individuals with whom I shared my time and talents in service as a pianist and singer. When given the cold shoulder, I realized I was expendable. I recognized that the love of many was conditional.

The feelings of rejection that welled up in me produced mental bugs that made me question my place in God's creation. I wondered if I were meant to be part of the True Vine. Bugs will spread and swarm, invading branches, stunting growth, or causing death. Allowing any "bugs" to live in us limits our capacity to bear fruit and impacts the life of every other branch, every other person. So the idea of compromising someone else's ability to grow or heal prompted me to do some "pruning."

I worked to eliminate thoughts that demeaned my identity. I spent time figuring out what kept me from being my truest self. I addressed the internalized phobias that shamed being trans and bisexual or queer. I unpacked the confusion of being attracted to genders both the same and different from mine, which can prove confusing and flustering (if you let it). I unlearned—I am unlearning!—toxic traits about being a man, which is an identity I was conditioned to assume but one that did not align with me.

Having to shake off the attacks on my blackness, whether that be comments about the hue of my skin or the tone of my voice (which was said to not be black enough, whatever that means), being questioned for possessing a certain level of intelligence counter to what my classmates saw portrayed in media, I resolved that I did not have to fit a mold to qualify as Black. Black persons are not monolithic and therefore are allowed to not act in the same way but still maintain their blackness without a critique to identity.

Womanism helped liberate my closeted self, inviting me to live into a wholeness and authenticity that the Divine One has for me. Coined by author Alice Walker, Womanism springs from the intersectional experiences of Black women. Womanism named the elements of my upbringing that I tried to deny for the sake of living into an identity as a man that I could not uphold. It gave me the freedom to embrace not only the teachings of the Black women that nurtured me, but the feminine wisdom that moves through me. I embrace my call to care, and I am learning how to balance this call with healthy boundaries.

I am finding ways to abide in God and abide in community. While I know that *I* am not the issue that people need to wrestle with, I still become the target for their confusion, frustration, or dismissal. Some days it becomes difficult to serve in ministry when parts of the community fail to recognize or respect a level of difference that they cannot understand or refuse to understand. Recognizing that we are all on a journey, I try to practice grace in a way that preserves my choice to be authentic while supporting someone else's journey of understanding and processing new information. It's fine to be hopeful and want change to occur overnight but being realistic reminds me that it may take a while for someone to see the Imago Dei in me when they did not know the Imago Dei can exist in this form. Their lack of recognition does not negate my ability to see God in them.

We must be committed to each other's flourishing—not just survival—and this requires connection. I love sharing that I am a fourth generation Disciple. My home church, Second Christian Church, is over 150 years old. My mom, aunts, and cousins filled positions as ushers, committee chairs, cooks, musicians, deacons, and elders. I grew up cutting my teeth on the pews and learned how to respond to the sermonic cadence of my pastor, Rev. M. Faye Vaughn, shouting "amen!" with the rest of the congregation. I sang in the youth choir at the age of four and by twelve years old I became a part-time pianist for my church. This church continues to claim me as a child of the village.

Maybe Gilbert Baker assigned sunlight to the color yellow for its ability to foster and nourish growth. For me this translates to bodies, specifically but not exclusively queer bodies deserving affirmation. When some in our community were told that they deserved to perish, the sunlight was a ray of hope that shouted otherwise.

You need sunlight to make rainbows in the sky. There's something about water crystals needed to make a rainbow...but the arc of colors is illumined by the sunlight flowing through.

Basking in its warm glow, let us pass on the warmth of sunlight through actions that motivate others to grow. May we support one another, cling to the True Vine, and prune anything that deadens our branches or spoils our fruit. I have a few experiences of this warming sunlight, of supportive actions from others that helped me grow.

When serving an Episcopal church as its choirmaster and organist, I began to give myself permission to ease out of a masculine identity. I explored my understanding of the feminine through decorative expressions on my body. Excited by different hues and shades of color, I found myself drawn to the sparkly eye shadow of a few parishioners, one of whom I spoke to and hugged every time we had a gathering. One day in the season of Advent, she wore a rose gold eye shadow that I complimented. We exchanged our usual hug, and she told me where she purchased the makeup.

Later in the month the parishioner placed a brown bag in my hands. With a warm smile on her face, she told me I would wear the eye shadow better than her. I disagreed but hugged her tightly and thanked her for the gift. While I don't need to dress a certain way to validate what a nonbinary person looks like, that gift of eye shadow affirmed my self-expression.

I acquired my first set of hoop earrings in that same parish. I admired a parishioner's earrings during the passing of the peace, and in the recessional line after the service, she placed in my hand two hoop earrings with a metal lace pattern. She told me to keep hold of them and wear them once I got my ears pierced. What she didn't know is that my love for hoop earrings stems from watching my mother pop off with style, dawning at least one gold hoop for her nights out with friends; Mother doesn't like to match her earrings. The earrings not only affirmed my gender exploration but invited me to enjoy the same affection for earrings that my mother possessed—and maybe passed on to me. I suppose it's in our family tree!

> Who the Sun sets free is free to be
>
> Glittering, shining, basking in amber warmth
>
> Rays on rays on rays of endless paths
>
> Dancing across the sky in ribbons
>
> Inviting, it calls for you
>
> Inviting, it dares you to

See the one whose hue

Shares a lil dandelion color too.

Under this same Sun we are invited to interact with one another in thought, word, and deed, strengthening our relationships and expanding our web of connection with all of creation. Beguiled by the sun's morning tapestry and blessed by its evening golden-hour filter, we all get a little extra sparkle. Hoop earrings or not.

May you rise in the glow of the sun, be immersed in its golden goodbye, and find rest and renewal in the shade of the night.

Amen and Ase.

Wonder

In this season of your life, do you desire deeper connection with God or with community?

Do you need sunlight, shade or pruning?

Resist

The author writes, "recognizing that we are all on a journey, I try to practice grace in a way that preserves my choice to be authentic while supporting someone else's journey of understanding and processing new information..." In what ways might you be called to "practice grace"?

Embody

How are you harnessing the warmth of sunlight? Find ways throughout your day to emulate the warmth or recognize actions that produce a similar feeling.

Observe the color yellow and use its vibrancy to energize the start of your day.

Create

The author opens their devotion with prose, "As the Earth rotates…" and closes with a poem, "Who the Sun sets free…"

Create your own prose or poetry about the sun.

Hope

The author reminds us that we share an abundant resource. What would it mean to live in a world where everyone has enough?

Dream and envision how we can share resources.

Stretch

Stretch your mind: are you familiar with Womanism? Do some research. Record what you learn.

Stretch your creativity: Go on a scavenger hunt and collect anything yellow. At the end of your adventure, arrange your pieces into a work of art and take a picture. Write about your experience, give your art a title, and provide a description as if it were displayed in a museum.

Share

While it likely won't look like gifts of eye shadow or hoop earrings, how can you "pass on the warmth of sunlight through actions that motivate others to grow"?

But maybe: Is there a gift (handmade or otherwise) that you can share?

And how have you experienced this "warming sunlight"?

Green + Nature

Every Body

Melissa Guthrie (she/her)

O sing to the LORD a new song,
  for he has done marvelous things.
His right hand and his holy arm
  have gotten him victory.
The LORD has made known his victory;
  he has revealed his vindication in the sight of the nations.
He has remembered his steadfast love and faithfulness
  to the house of Israel.
All the ends of the earth have seen
  the victory of our God.

Make a joyful noise to the LORD, all the earth;
  break forth into joyous song and sing praises.
Sing praises to the LORD with the lyre,
  with the lyre and the sound of melody.
With trumpets and the sound of the horn
  make a joyful noise before the King, the LORD.

Let the sea roar, and all that fills it;
  the world and those who live in it.
Let the floods clap their hands;
  let the hills sing together for joy
at the presence of the LORD, for he is coming
  to judge the earth.
He will judge the world with righteousness,
  and the peoples with equity. (Psalm 98)

I wanted to sit outside, by the stream, among the trees. *In* "nature." The pollen was thick though. And every, every single neighbor seemed to be mowing or blowing leaves. Sounds of construction—destruction?—these noises filled my outdoors.

I need sunlight. And yellow is one of my two favorite colors. My other favorite is not green but pink. Wanting to be *out* in the yard, on the lawn furniture because I love nature but don't like bugs, I settled for sitting in the soft yellow rays of the day's sunlight streaming through my living room window. "Dog poop!" my toddler screams, interrupting my sunlit serenity. She was outside the front door and had either stepped in it or—I hope not!—scooped it up. I yelled at my wife, "I'm trying to write about nature in here!"

My wife (thinks she) is funny. She responded, "Everybody poops. It's a natural part of life."

I suppose "shift happens." I did say shift…

Wanting to distance myself from "the shift that happens" and shift back to my work and writing, I imagined myself on a sandy beach listening to the sea roar. Then I saw myself on a snow-capped mountain scaling its peak.

Since the sunlit dog poop incident, I've traveled to the beach and the mountains. At the beach I listened to the sea roar and a group of kids complain about the heat and sand. In the mountains, I hiked serene trails to escape and walked busy streets to shop. My senses absorbed the autumn colors, cool temperatures, and tree songs. You know, the tree song is a subtle rustle with heightened whispers from the wind. It's conversation between the leaves. The trees tell secrets!

I swear the leaves on the maple tree turned a richer orange as I blinked; the leaves were entertaining me with a dance recital and swift costume changes. "Look at my gifts," they prided; gloriously green and red and orange and yellow. And rust and mauve and cabernet sauvignon. I had a fall wedding because I love these colors. The bridal party asked, "What color red do you want us to wear?" "Not red," I said. "The rich color of a really good Cab." *That color.*

At Christmount, a retreat, camp, and conference center of the Christian Church (Disciples of Christ) in Black Mountain, North Carolina, I took in the sounds of a nearby stream, birds, and a rooster—where was that rooster?—as well as church bells, highway traffic, and more leaf blowing. *Does everyone everywhere blow leaves when I just want to be? Let the leaves be! Let me be.* There was silence and banter between kids, plus bickering between family members. I admired thin silver threads of a spider web stretched between the slats of a rocking chair, and I enjoyed the string lights on the porch. The sun warmed my shoulders and made my laptop too hot.

Do you see it and experience it too?

The "natural environment" blurs with the "built environment." We tend to think of nature as "out there" and "apart from" us. We go out into nature. But what if, what if nature is not (only) "out there"?

Nature, wilderness, environment—those terms don't hold universal meaning. Our ideas about what constitutes "nature" or the "natural" and "unnatural" are completely bound up in our personal histories and cultural assumptions. The natural environment is also a built environment, one shaped by and experienced through assumptions and expectations about ability, gender, sexuality, class, race, and nation.

Having used Alison Kafer's book *Feminist, Queer, Crip*[9] in a divinity school course on theology and disability, I revisited her chapter titled "Bodies of Nature: The Environmental Politics of Disability." Kafer questions our assumptions and expectations related to the environment. And Kafer suggests "person" and "plant" are not so easily distinguished. I think of "the world and its inhabitants" in Psalm 98. With the lyre and trumpets, with the sea thundering, rivers clapping and mountains singing, the world and its inhabitants make quite a noise. There's a swirl, a blur of human and nonhuman song.

Years before reading Kafer, I founded the faith-rooted nonprofit Salvage Garden. *We're not a gardening club.* Salvage Garden strives to reclaim the value of all individuals; its primary offering is "The Banquet," a multi-sensory worship experience for all ages and all abilities. When the community gathers for worship, the people speak in (attempted) unison: "We come from different places with different stories. We celebrate the diversity of our human family and the unity

---

[9]Alison Kafer, *Feminist, Queer, Crip* (Bloomington, IN: Indiana University Press, 2013).

of our call to love and justice. We are God's people. We belong to God and we belong to each other."

The juxtaposition of "salvage" and "garden" is significant, as is our artwork. How to describe the logo for Salvage Garden? Drawing upon renderings of the Tree of Life, a divinity school colleague Christine Hargraves created a banner that depicts both a salvage yard and a garden with "SG" smoothly blended into the leaves and branches of a large tree. In the banner: "tree people" or "people that grow." You'll have to see Salvage Garden's artwork. Person and plant are not so easily distinguished.

"Tree people" from Salvage Garden? "Rivers clapping and mountains singing" in the Psalm? That's not normal...That's not natural...Queer siblings and allies, how often do we hear, "that's not natural!?!"

I treasure the immensity and diversity of Creation, all bodies of nature. Through the ministries of Salvage Garden and AllianceQ – the Disciples LGBTQ+ Alliance, I've devoted most of my professional work to reclaiming the value of every body, bodies inextricably connected to one another and with nature. I'm GLAD to work with ministries that affirm our divine differences.

Kafer and the psalmist and—surprise—Gilbert Baker invite us to reimagine how we understand ourselves and our bodies in relationship to nature. We are interdependent. Every body is a vital part of the landscape. Every body is in; no one excluded. No one "left out." Also, please "come out" if you're not living fully as your divinely created self. Gender, sexuality, ability...joy, grief, togetherness, brokenness...All of you is entirely marvelous. And we need not be bound to binaries: natural or unnatural, nature and self. God and creation: *much too expansive.*

"O sing to the LORD a new song, for he has done marvelous things...Make a joyful noise to the LORD, all the earth; break forth..."

In Psalm 98, praise for the Creator blasts from horns; praise roars from the sea and the fish and coral reefs. Praise for the Creator cannot be contained. We cannot contain or explain the marvelous things the Lord has done. Still, we rationalize, explain away, "water down" the fullness of the Divine. Or we withhold our song.

It's personification. Hyperbole. Metaphor.

The hills don't sing—*do they?* Imagine if they did. The rivers don't clap, but imagine if they did. Imagine if we, with all the earth and its inhabitants, made a joyful noise: a just noise for all humankind on a thriving earth. Do you sing when your soul is happy? Do you sing when your soul needs freedom? Do you listen to your sibling's song and the tree's song?

Here I (re)turn to Gilbert Baker's green stripe. It is said that nature sat at the core of Baker's movement. From the San Francisco Green Film Festival's explanation of the colors of the Pride flag:

> The beauty of pride—celebrating love, humanity, and acceptance of and for everybody—is intrinsically tied with nature. To openly express and share one's sexuality is natural. To be gay, lesbian, bisexual, queer, or transgender is natural. To love and be loved by others is natural. Our earth, its resources, its healing and feeding capabilities, are all apart [sic] of the pride movement's overarching goals for peace, love, and equality. For humans and the planet earth alike.[10]

All a part of the movement. With the raucous in you and around you, know that you—your body, your love, your joy, your grief—all of you is affirmed and connected with the whole of God's creation.

Because we are interdependent, how do we care for God's creation? I'm moved by this covenant from Green Chalice, part of the missions and advocacy with Disciples Home Missions:

> As children of God and followers of Christ Jesus, we covenant to:
>
> Worship God with all creation and pray for the healing of the earth.
>
> Study the climate crisis and engage others in climate solutions.
>
> Repent and forgive for the harm we have inflicted on the earth that sustains life.
>
> Advocate for ecojustice public policies and witness by living sustainable lifestyles.

---

[10] "The Green Stripe," https://www.greenfilmfest.org/thegreenstripe.

Rest in God's good creation and invite others to delight in nature.[11]

Growing up, I delighted in nature and I despaired about the planet. I gave my mom a lot of grief. I'm sure she would say I made an awful lot of annoying noise. Not sure when or why it struck me so deeply. I cared especially about the birds of the air. If my mom threw her chewing gum out the car window, I pleaded for her to pull over and pick up the gum. I belabored my point, "The birds will get it and choke on it and die!" I've since learned that birds rarely die from ingesting gum. But trash has negative effects on the environment, which ultimately affects birds.

I have a tattoo of a dove; in its mouth is a rose. I have a favorite poem about a rose opening in its own time. But I suppose the bird needs bubble gum in its beak! A tattooed dove with bubble gum in its beak would connect all my stories: my story of self, my relationships with others (especially my mother), and creation. By the way, my mom stopped throwing out her gum, and I'm not redoing my tattoo. But what body art will I get next? My mom doesn't like tattoos. (I love you, Mom!)

From the Psalms to the gospels, from our faith communities to the streets of every city, the beaches to the plains to cornfields and mountain peaks, may we embrace and honor our place in God's love story. May we celebrate love, humanity, and acceptance of and for everybody. May we strive for peace, love, and equality. For humans (and birds) and the planet Earth alike. *Thanks, Baker, for weaving us and all the colors together.*

The psalmist invites us to sing. You should sing. I should sing. I should sing alone. Or in the shower or in the car. Singing is not one of my spiritual gifts; even so, even more, I'll make a joyful noise. With all the earth, may we sing a new song, praising a creator who, Psalm 98, verse 9, a creator who will rule the world justly, and its people with equity.

Please don't throw your gum on the ground. And I hope you don't step in dog poop.

I invite you to pray with your body. Touch your bare feet to the street,

---

[11]"Green Chalice Covenant," https://www.discipleshomemissions.org/missions-advocacy/green-chalice/green-chalice-covenant-2/.

the sand, or the grass. Roll your wheelchair to a space near the trees. With the palm of your hand feel the bark of a tree. However your body experiences the world, take in all the noise, all the colors, and connect your breath to the wind.

You are a vital part of the landscape.

Amen.

Wonder

What's your definition of "nature," "wilderness," "environment"?

How have you come to understand "natural" and "unnatural"? Spend time exploring your assumptions and expectations. How have your beliefs been built?

Resist

How can you contribute to the thriving of our earth?

What can you reduce or eliminate to be eco-friendly?

Embody

When have you felt connected with the earth?

Spend time (more time than usual) outdoors. What does this feel like for your body? Mind? Spirit?

Plant something. Eat a locally sourced food. Prepare an entire meal with homegrown or locally grown ingredients.

Create

How do you express praise for the Creator?

Compose your very own "praise song."

Listen to praise songs. Listen to songs about creation.

Hope

The author says we are interdependent and asks how we care for God's creation, "the world and those who live in it." How does our interconnectedness prompt despair and/or give you hope?

List some of the "marvelous things God has done."

Revisit your "praise song." Do you sing praise for these marvelous things?

Stretch

The author references a book chapter, "Bodies of Nature." Find a book or resource about the body and/or nature to expand your understanding of one or both.

Can you imagine blurring the distinctions between "person" and "plant"? Write about or illustrate what comes to mind.

Share

Examine your own practices and/or the practices of your faith community and commit to three changes that will move you toward better caring for God's creation. What are your three changes?

Tell someone about your commitment so you have accountability. Who did you tell? How did that conversation go?

Who can you invite to do likewise?

Turquoise + Art/Magic

A (Magical) Work of Art

Renair Amin (she/they)

Then Moses said to the Israelites: See, the LORD has called by name Bezalel son of Uri son of Hur, of the tribe of Judah; he has filled him with divine spirit, with skill, intelligence, and knowledge in every kind of craft, to devise artistic designs, to work in gold, silver, and bronze, in cutting stones for setting, and in carving wood, in every kind of craft. And he has inspired him to teach, both him and Oholiab son of Ahisamach, of the tribe of Dan. He has filled them with skill to do every kind of work done by an artisan or by a designer or by an embroiderer in blue, purple, and crimson yarns, and in fine linen, or by a weaver—by any sort of artisan or skilled designer. (Exodus 35:30–35)

Often when people think of art their minds go to some of the greatest artists of all time. Michelangelo. Baldwin. Picasso. Basquiat. No matter the medium, art engages our emotions and prompts self-reflection. What is art? Most people reference something from this list: painting, sculpture, literature, cinema, music, theatre, photography, digital art, and architecture. Architecture is what we have in the Exodus passage, well, Bezalel has "knowledge in every kind of craft."

The beauty—and sometimes the challenge—is that you decide what constitutes art. Critics and intellectuals and parents of small children who make "art" have debated this for centuries. For me, it's nature. And I think God is the Master Artist.

At a retreat site outside Atlanta, Georgia, where I was facilitating a workshop, I needed a quiet place to gather my thoughts. I enjoyed a walk down to the lake on the other side of the campground. Sitting by the lake, I was moved to tears as I admired the sun rise over the trees. It was as if the whole world was waking up. The artistry of the sunrise seemed...magical. I walked to that spot every day, absorbing something new each time. Almost ten years later, I have the video that I recorded my last day there. I watch the video occasionally; it reminds me to see the sun even on my cloudiest days.

When life does what life does, it can be hard to see the sun through the clouds. Our minds fill with worry or negativity. In some cases, depression ensues. In others, a trauma response sets in, and we find ourselves in places of fight-or-flight. In our darkest hours, we may hope for a light at the end of the tunnel. In the tunnel or at the end of the tunnel, many find inspiration. In fact, pain is often the catalyst to creative expression.

My deepest pains have inspired my greatest works. I have written books about surviving intimate partner violence, tragedy, and broken relationships. As far back as my childhood, I remember writing acrostic poems after a disagreement with my mom. Just a few months ago, I found a journal written at the end of my marriage. I risked rereading the pages, remembering my state when I poured my pain on the pages. It was interesting to look back on a period that at the time felt like an end, but turns out it was a new beginning. I am not the only artist that has been able to transmute their pain into something powerful.

Throughout history we find individuals who chose art to help process the trauma in their lives. For example, sculptor Rodin created "The Kiss" and "The Eternal Idol" after a romantic split from a fellow artist. Painter Francis Bacon produced "In Memory of George Dyer" after the death of his partner. Rita O'Hara found relief through her art after being diagnosed with rheumatoid arthritis. As a person who lives with inflammatory arthritis, this was inspiring to me!

There is something powerful about taking a situation and looking at it through another lens. You almost become an alchemist of your own life by transforming something through a seemingly magical process. Have you ever seen a work of art and wondered how the artist was able to create it? Have you ever heard someone's story and thought to yourself, "How are they still standing?" Their resilience and the beauty of their story stir something deep within you.

Have you experienced a tumultuous season that served as a catalyst for some creative expression? Have you ever been charged to lead a project in the midst of chaos? Have you been called to encourage and inspire the people in your life through what you create? Yes, you are an artist of your own kind! Let's look at the chief artisan in the Exodus passage that describes the preparations for construction of the Tabernacle.

Bezalel was called by God to build the tabernacle as well as the ark of the covenant. This assignment was given after the Israelites were punished for asking Aaron to build them a golden calf to worship when they feared their leader Moses was not returning from Mount Sinai. Fear. Fight-or-flight. Moses informed the people of God's command and Bezalel set out to fulfill his call. Once everything was set up and consecrated for use, God's presence appeared as a cloud and descended on the tabernacle. From that day forward, God would appear in the form of a cloud to indicate that Israel was to move camp.

The Israelites were moving on from a catastrophic moment in their journey, reclaiming their covenant with God. How amazing is that! Despite their past, once they were able to get back in alignment in their relationship with God, the trajectory shifted. They were once again in a place to move in their Purpose.

This would not have been possible without the lead engineer Bezalel. Yes, one may argue that the task could have been completed without him, but it would not have been the same. When you are moving in your Purpose, there is only one you. Your presence is needed for the Work and all the people meant to experience your influence.

Although Moses and the people approved of Bezalel being lead on the construction of the tabernacle, it was God who called him. It is important to remember that others cannot stop you from doing what God has deemed for you to do in your life. Even if you experience a detour along the way, you learn a lesson from the situation and move forward in your journey. An old saying goes, "a delay is not a denial." We see this in the story of the Israelites.

Bezalel embraced the gifts placed in him to lead the project, and he was made a teacher to share his skills with others. The "teachings" we receive are not just to help us design a better life for ourselves but to empower others. Through our testimonies and lived examples, others glean how to do similar Work in their lives. Whether it is the development of a tangible skill or a new way of being, our lives can become a (magical) work of art. And people will want to know how you were able to create it. People often see the finished product; you get to share how the art emerged.

I did not always share my stories. Growing up, I was encouraged to keep my life private. My mom was a stickler on not allowing any family business to leave the house. I made a strong effort to not give others access to what was happening in my life—and this would eventually lead to my detriment. At the age of twelve, I was assaulted and felt like I could not—no, should not—tell anyone including my mom. I lived in pain until I turned eighteen years old and finally confided in my mom.

I would still pick and choose with whom I shared my journey. Until I resumed writing poetry. I met another poet who encouraged me to perform on stage at an open mic event she was organizing. When the time came, I flew from Philadelphia, Pennsylvania, to Rochester, New York, and presented my first spoken word piece. I remember one lady coming up to me after the show, telling me that my poem spoke to her, that she could relate to my experience. This changed my life. From that point forward, I shared my story any way I could and still do. Each time, I am reminded how I overcame challenges. I revisit lessons learned.

Sharing your lessons learned and the steps in your process proves helpful because it may have taken more than one footstep to arrive at your place of healing. Perhaps you didn't know that you possessed the skills. The Word says that Bezalel was given the skills to do every kind of work. God knew what Bezalel needed to bring to life the tabernacle. God knows what you need to move to your next destination.

The Word says that Bezalel was filled with wisdom and knowledge. It is one thing to be taught a skill. It is another to have the wisdom to apply what is learned. Navigating life requires skills and wisdom. Keeping a journal helps me garner some wisdom from life. I can reshape my story and forge appreciation for and understanding of the good and bad (and really good and really bad) experiences. All of which becomes influential as I build—as you build—the masterpieces that are our lives.

What will go into your showpiece? You get to choose the medium. And the colors. What textures and elements will tell your story? For instance, you could use red to show passion or green to show prosperity. When Gilbert Baker included the turquoise color in the Pride flag, it represented art and magic. Although turquoise and pink are no longer part of Baker's Pride flag due to manufacturing costs, the colors portray an important part of history from the LGBTQ+ movement.

Baker chose turquoise to epitomize the LGBTQ+ artists who were using their creative expressions to challenge discrimination. Whether it was poet activist Audre Lorde breaking down walls of injustice or disco singer Sylvester redefining the binary, their art changed the world. I think it is profound that Gilbert Baker included turquoise and art in the Pride flag, highlighting the brilliance of LGBTQ+ art as activism. It's just magical.

The greatest artists evoke some personal and collective change.

I want to watch my decade-old video of the sunrise. And I want to absorb each morning's sunrise. I want to wake up with the world and make art.

The Lord called Bezalel, and you, and me by name; he has filled us with divine spirit, with skill, intelligence, and knowledge in every kind of craft...and has inspired us to teach...

Bezalel was able to emerge from a tumultuous time in a way that helped people enhance their lives and reestablish their relationships with God. The way he moved in his Purpose honored God, and everyone got to see the fruits of his learning. What are your gifts? What is it that you want to design for your life? What can you draw from your past or current experiences to help you in the future? What can you share from your story to help others create works of art?

Yes, you are an artist. Maybe not a tabernacle architect. But you are an artist. And your life is a (magical) work of art.

Wonder

What is art?

What types of art do you appreciate?

The author said she sees nature as art. What "art" do you see in nature?

Resist

The author says she was encouraged to keep her life private and that led to her detriment. Are there any expectations of you that you recognize you should resist?

Embody

Think about your favorite work of art or select a work that represents you. Explain why you selected the work or how the art represents you.

Do you have any body art? Tattoos, piercings or other? (There's a range of body art...)

Thoughts about body art?

Create

Are you a traditional artist? What art can you experiment with or what craft can you learn?

Hope

What is your desire for the masterpiece that is your life?

If there were no obstacles in the way, how would your life look? Feel free to envision your greatest dream. After you are done, reread it and bask in the feeling of your "life" as if you are currently living it. (Note: Feel free to revisit what you have written daily or at least once a week to keep you inspired about the life you are looking to create.)

Stretch

The author writes, "...an alchemist transforms or creates something through a seemingly magical process. Have you ever seen a work of art and wondered how the artist was able to create it? Have you ever heard someone's story and thought to yourself, 'How are they still standing?'"

Do you know someone who is "still standing"? If yes, how was that person resilient?

If there is a tumultuous situation in your life or the life of a loved one, how will you transmute your pain or support the loved one?

Share

Reflect on the skills Bezalel possessed and what those skills meant to his community. Write down your insights.

Consider the skills, knowledge, or wisdom you possess. Make a list.

How can those things be helpful to your community? (Note: Your community may be family, friends, or external connections.) Identify one skill to share in a new way. When will you share this skill?

Blue + Harmony/Serenity

Seeing with Spiritual Eyes

Brendan Y. Boone (he/him)

The LORD is my shepherd, I shall not want.
He makes me lie down in green pastures;
he leads me beside still waters;
he restores my soul.
He leads me in right paths
for his name's sake. (Psalm 23:1–3)

Whenever you entered the homes of our mother and aunt (fondly known as "Auntie" to many), there were at least three things you could count on seeing hanging somewhere near the entrance, in the living room, or in the bedroom: The Lord's Prayer, Psalm 23, or The Ten Commandments. And a rendering of the church we were raised in at some point in our lives. Our aunt also had a picture of Jesus which hung on the wall over her bed. You may remember seeing those writings, etched in red on a white porcelain plate, complete with a metal hanger, so it could be displayed in a prominent place for all to see. We have three of the plates hanging in our home office now.

Over the years, I have come to believe Mother and Auntie displayed these Christian symbols as a way of expressing their faith, claiming God's protection over their homes and all who entered, and communicating to friends and guests that, as Joshua proclaimed many centuries ago, "now if you are unwilling to serve the LORD, choose this day whom you will serve...but as for me and my household, we will serve the LORD" (Joshua 24:15). They were God-fearing and God-loving women who always started and ended their days in meditation and prayer. Even as arthritis and two amputations took its toll on our mother's body and dementia would eventually rob our aunt of her cognitive abilities, they never forgot about family, God, the name of Jesus, the power of prayer, or the capacity to genuinely love, pray for and respect others. They dedicated their whole lives to serving God by serving others in whatever ways they could. God was without question their Shepherd, and while we did not have a lot, we did not have a need God did not meet.

> *"GOD, my Shepherd! I don't need a thing. You have bedded me down in lush meadows, you find me quiet pools to drink from. True to Your word, You let me catch my breath and send me in the right direction." (Psalm 23:1–3, The Message)*

As a "second generation" child for my mother, she relied heavily on my "other mother" Auntie, as well as a community of women from the church and neighborhood to help raise, look out for, and care for me while she worked as a nurse to support the two of us and my sister who had just started college. As the church, and more importantly, my "adopted mothers" would start to learn about me as a same-gender loving person (although no one ever asked me directly), they still embraced me. Even when I would return to the church from time to time as the person I have always known myself to be, they still welcomed me, loved me, encouraged me, and inquired about me and my life.

It would be in this community of faith I would learn the importance of seeing others with spiritual eyes. These are the saints who would significantly influence and help shape an integral part of my spiritual foundation for which I am eternally grateful. This community of faith served as the place where I would come to understand the importance of striving to live a life rooted in peace and creating an environment where harmony and unity are both encouraged and embraced. This continual quest for internal peace and harmony is one of the many reasons I love going to the beach.

In the mid to late 1970s, after my first end-of-summer recreation trip to Ocean View Amusement Park and the beach, I developed a deep love of the beach. While I am not a swimmer, the beach continues to be my "go-to" when I just need to get away from it all, sit, breathe, and be. With the blue skies as my canopy, I love listening to the sound of the ocean waves crashing on the shore, feeling the warmth of the sand on my feet and in between my toes, and walking through the water along the seashore. It is a new experience every time I go.

To exhale the stress of days past and reflect on current realities while taking in the magnificent wonder of God's creative signature upon the earth is a balm to my soul. Amid the noise and chatter of all the surrounding beachgoers and sun worshippers, there is a simple serenity that envelopes my soul and spirit, inviting me to just let go and let God. It was as if the Spirit of God invited me to come and experience respite for my mind, body, and soul, being open to receive an inward renewal only God can offer and provide through "quiet pools to drink from."

Every visit to the beach affords me an opportunity to learn something more about God and about myself. Whether you are at the beach, out in the ocean, or on the lake there is so much to learn from the natural environment. Such an opportunity presented itself many years ago while on vacation at the beach. Having a whole week gave me an abundance of time to spend at the ocean's edge.

Watching the waves wash up on the shoreline, the ocean waters showed a greenish tint. When I was younger, I assumed the ocean water was green, not realizing at that age there was so much more to the ocean than what I was seeing with my human eyes. It would be on my first boat ride a little further out into open waters where the color would gradually become blue, stretching further than the eye could see. Fascinated by what I was seeing, I spent most of my time on the boat looking at the water, absorbing the richness of the colors. The more I watched the water, the more I felt drawn in. While no one could "see" me having this experience, there was an internal feeling unfolding: peace. During those holy moments on that boat, I was able to see the water from a distinct perspective and experience it in new ways using what I like to call my "spiritual eyes." Simply put, to see with spiritual eyes is to see beyond what the human eye can see, seeking what is invisible or underneath the veneer.

Prior to that moment, I really did not pay much attention to the diverse hues and tones all around us. My experiences at the beach and on the water invited me to be aware of the color palette around me and pay attention to how I emotionally and physiologically respond to the various shades. Just as colors can represent things like seasons in the church's liturgical calendar, objects, people, moments in time and history, movement, and the like, colors have the capacity to elicit emotional responses, some visible, others experienced within. Blue is a color known to generate emotional responses.

Each color of Gilbert Baker's flag was selected to represent some aspect of the LGBTQ+ community and blue expressed—or called for—harmony and serenity. While some may find it a bit odd (a color representing an emotion or feeling), the blue stripe was essential. In the early days of the movement, our ancestors fought relentlessly for justice, equality, and inclusion, often putting themselves and their lives on the line—in some cases, losing their lives. In some way, those on the frontlines of the movement needed a visual aid to remind them they were individuals within a larger collective. There could be and would be harmony and serenity within themselves and the world. Also, a movement can only be as healthy as the members within it. To be aware of and care for one's personal well-being was essential. Blue was included among the rainbow colors as a reminder of personal wellness and community wellness. Individuals and groups both need periods of rest and restoration, as well as physical, emotional, and spiritual regeneration.

Blue has a place in the biblical witness as well, beginning with the very creation of the heavens and earth. From a spiritual perspective, blue is understood to represent the presence and healing power of God. In both the Hebrew and Christian Testaments, blue is present in a variety of ways. In Numbers 15: 38–39, the children of Israel were instructed to "make fringes on the corners of their garments throughout their generations and to put a blue cord on the fringe at each corner. You have the fringe so that, when you see it, you will remember all the commandments of the LORD and do them, and not follow the lust of your own heart and your own eyes." In the story of the woman with the issue of blood, she believed if she could touch the hem of Jesus' garment, she would be made whole (Matthew 9). The hem of Jesus' garment was believed to be blue.

From a human perspective, blue can be a catalyst for generating several responses in the body. It can have a calming effect upon a person when the body releases chemicals intended to provide a sense of relief in the body. Blue is known to aid in one's productivity and enhance intuitive abilities. Interestingly, while blue is often associated with a woman giving birth to a baby boy, the color itself is thought to be less specific in terms of gender. Many people across the gender spectrum prefer blue as a color. This certainly makes a case for opening the circle of humanity wider, ensuring nonbinary and gender nonconforming persons are included. If you spend any time watching TV during the evening hours, pay attention to commercials advertising various sleep or calming aids. A vast majority of the commercials are promoting products...in some sort of blue package! There is something alluring and relaxing about the color blue.

The desire and need for internal peace and a hope for unity and harmony seem to be the order of the day for most. Amid life struggles, the relentless presence of a pandemic and a feeling of disconnection from those who are near and dear to us, there is a need for a spiritual reset to reclaim a sense of balance and clarity. Should we make time to spend with God in prayer and meditation, we can refocus and begin to see things, ourselves, and others differently. It is about learning to see with spiritual eyes and allowing God through the Spirit to lead.

The Spirit may lead you to the beach. If so, I'll be there, with Psalm 23 on my mind and Mother and Auntie and all the saints in harmony with us.

Wonder

Who are the spiritual influencers in your life and in what ways did they contribute to your spiritual foundation and growth?

If you could send them a note or letter, what would you say to them? Journal about this and as you feel comfortable, share your thoughts with someone. (Or send that note!)

Resist

Where is your "go-to" place to refresh, rest, and renew? What makes this location the ideal place for you? What are the various emotions and feelings you experience while there?

Hope as an act of resistance requires our self-care. How do you resist burnout?

Embody

Do you have access to a lake, river, creek, the ocean, or a swimming pool? Take yourself there! What colors do you see on the surface and then below? Pay attention to all your senses. What are you experiencing?

Unable to access one of these bodies of water? Fill a bowl with water.

Outdoors or indoors, touch the water with your hands or toes. (Or go swimming!)

Create

What color would you most identify with as a reminder to seek harmony and serenity? In what ways can you begin to incorporate that color in your surroundings? Develop a plan which allows time for you to map out what this will look like and how it can happen.

How will you "open the circle of humanity wider," creating harmony beyond your own circle?

Hope

The author said his mother and auntie "dedicated their whole lives to serving God by serving others in whatever ways they could. God was, without question, their Shepherd, and while we did not have a lot, we did not have a need God did not meet." In what ways has the Shepherd met your needs?

Wherever the Spirit leads, how will you practice "seeing with spiritual eyes"?

Stretch

How will you "see" the color blue differently? If blue is viewed as a color embraced across the gender spectrum, what are some of the thought processes and assumptions that need to be challenged? Share your thoughts with someone.

Share

The author believes his mother and auntie displayed The Lord's Prayer, Psalm 23, and The Ten Commandments to express their faith. What symbols serve as displays of your faith?

Gather a small group of trusted friends. Share with them how the blue devotion or another devotion has been helpful.

Purple + Spirit

How else than by the Spirit

Allen V. Harris (he/him)

I have made your name known to those whom you gave me from the world. They were yours, and you gave them to me, and they have kept your word. Now they know that everything you have given me is from you; for the words that you gave to me I have given to them, and they have received them and know in truth that I came from you; and they have believed that you sent me. I am asking on their behalf; I am not asking on behalf of the world, but on behalf of those whom you gave me, because they are yours. All mine are yours, and yours are mine; and I have been glorified in them. And now I am no longer in the world, but they are in the world, and I am coming to you. Holy Father, protect them in your name that you have given me, so that they may be one, as we are one. (John 17:6–11)

Purple is one of my favorite colors. My favorite book as a child was *Harold and the Purple Crayon.* I've got tattoos with purple in them. Even my favorite preaching folder that I used for fourteen years at Franklin Circle Christian Church in Cleveland, Ohio, was a bright, brilliant purple. For some reason the color purple represents the Holy Spirit to me: audacious and bold and overflowing with power and love.

Spirit is my favorite facet of the Divine. The Holy Spirit functions as an intimate, perceptive, and cherished persona of the Holy Trinity in my spiritual life. I wish we had a holy quadinity because then Sophia could give us two feminine aspects of God. But Spirit it is. Now, if you had known me as a child, a youth, a young adult, you would never have guessed that I would one day be in love with this winsome, wily, and wonderful Holy Spirit. I was, by anybody's standards, an uptight, anal-retentive, anxious, tentative child. I always looked for the responses of others to see how I should act or feel or speak or even think. Who knows exactly why this was the case, but I believe it was in large part due to the absence of my father. My father had retired from the military to enjoy his young family, but then discovered he had cancer of the larynx. He died about three months before I was born.

I think other young children who have had a parent die, and maybe even children who are part of divorce, might have the same kinds of feelings. My father's death affected my sense of place in the world and my sense of self-identity and self-confidence. It would take much inner work, including years of therapy and the coaching of friends and mentors, to finally loosen up, to trust myself and not link my self-worth to other people's actions and views of me and to ultimately follow the winds of the Spirit. And follow the Spirit I did!

Somehow that wonderful Spirit emboldened me to come out as a gay man near the end of my seminary days. The Spirit coaxed me to follow the call to ministry that God had placed within me, ever more confident in the gifts and graces that others saw, and I discerned, within me. The Spirit even cajoled me to go to places that I vowed as a teenager I would never live, such as New York City and Washington, D.C.

The Spirit encouraged me to come out completely and unapologetically as a queer, same-gender-loving, sex-positive gay man and to remain steadfastly committed to being ordained, which I was. The Spirit counseled me then to seek every call I have followed comfortably and proudly (and vocally, as it was often noted). It was the Spirit, I do believe, that challenged me to address my white male privilege, and to be unabashedly feminist, anti-racist, and dedicated to justice and equity for persons who are transgender, nonbinary, differently-abled, or from a different economic, educational, social, or political background than me.

The Spirit motivated me to claim opportunities that all too often I was prohibited from accessing *and* move on from these very opportunities, to leave my achievements behind. I left the Senior Pastor position of Park Avenue Christian Church in New York City. I left the Senior Pastor position of Franklin Circle Christian Church in Cleveland,

Ohio. (I took my purple preaching folder with me!) I left the Regional Minister position of the Christian Church Capitol Area. In none of these instances was there necessarily a need to leave nor had anyone asked or intimated that I needed to move on. The Spirit called me deep inside and allowed me to understand that for the health and vitality of both the organizations of which I was a part and for me and my family, I needed to move on.

I recognize that as a white male who grew up in a middle class and educated household that I have privileges that were afforded to me that are not afforded to everybody. Likewise, I appreciate that there are those who feel the Spirit's call to move on but who cannot take the risks I have taken, who cannot leave without another position secured because of their circumstances and the limitations the world too often places on them because of their gender identity, age, race, sexual orientation, or abilities. I am humbled by this. Even so, I must acknowledge that there is within the very core of my being a reliance upon the Holy Spirit that remains a source of strength and courage and allows me to do significant risk-taking. Risk-seeking and risk-leaving.

In John 17:6–11, Jesus doesn't really mention "Spirit." One might think the text alongside Gilbert Baker's theme of spirit is not a good fit. One might think the better fit would be the section of the same "farewell discourse" when Jesus tells his disciples he is going to send the Holy Spirit, the Advocate and Comforter, after him. But no, the implications of the scripture burst with reliance upon the Spirit.

How else than by the Spirit's power could one explain Jesus having enough trust in this rag-tag band of disciples to leave in their care the future of all he had lived for, loved, and taught about? How else than by the Spirit's leading could Jesus be bold enough to encourage his followers to let go of all they have come to know to set out on a course that would change the world as they knew it? How else than by the Spirit's guidance could the disciples fathom a future without their teacher that would be greater than the past with him? The Spirit guides us in our risk-seeking and risk-leaving.

We often hear people say that we should "see the Christ in each other." This helps us honor one another and treat each other with respect and dignity. What if we also encouraged ourselves and others to see all people from God's vantage point? What if we brought the deep compassion, profound patience, and incredible hopefulness of the Divine Source of Life to every relationship in which we engage? And with ourselves first and foremost. Remembering how God sees us helps us claim the gifts of the Spirit more completely. The Spirit provokes us to perceive ourselves and others and the world in multiple ways and upside down, inside out ways!

This so very much reminds me of the kind of upside-down look that Alice Walker has in her book *The Color Purple*. I recall the moment where Celie says, "I think it pisses off God if you walk by the color purple in a field somewhere and don't notice it. People think pleasing God is all God cares about, but any fool living in the world can see it always trying to please us back." Spirit prompts us to notice. Spirit reorients our thinking. Spirit animates us with joy, confidence, and a new hope.

Following the Spirit, through therapy and through the care and love of people around me, I perceive my experiences in a new way. My father's death did not in fact leave me abandoned. My father had been in relationship with so many people who were still with me, my mother most especially. The people who surrounded me as a child passed on his care, wisdom, and love, along with their own care, wisdom, and love, as the disciples passed on to so many others who Jesus was to them. And others have come in their place to pass on care, wisdom, love, stories, empowerment, and courage. I am indebted to the people and relationships that have helped me see myself in a different way. Maybe even helped me see myself from God's perspective.

And eventually, in the way that often comes from life and inheritance and time, I discovered that I am the one who is passing on care, wisdom, and love. I'm trying my best to empower others to see themselves as God perceives them, and to not bypass the purple fields of their lives and fail to be in awe and wonder of their own gifts and graces. Knowing that we are cared for by others, by the divine, even when they are not physically present here, even when they are gone, as the disciples would when Jesus left, gives us a self-assurance and a willingness and readiness to make the daring and often risk-taking decisions that make new possibilities open within us and before us.

This is the work of the Holy Spirit, which reminds me of another favorite piece of literature. It is a poem about following the whims of the Spirit, of being so confident in your own skin, of being so abundantly in touch with how beautiful you are that you take risks you wouldn't have before. The piece happens to be one of the most notable poems about the color purple. You might not know it by its title or author, "Warning" by Jenny Joseph, but many will know it by its famous opening line, "When I am an old woman, I shall wear purple."

The poet describes in detail the way she might dress or eat or behave in public because of the confidence that she gains as she grows older; she is less and less worried about other people's opinions about how she acts and feels and speaks and even thinks. She surmises that this carefree life is so delightful she might need to start "practicing" right away how she will behave when she is old. Why? "So people who know me are not too shocked and surprised when suddenly I am old and start to wear purple."

Don't we want that same kind of confidence, and don't we want to practice that same kind of risk-taking, comfortable-in-our-own-skin selves, as young as we possibly can? For me, part of this is opening up the world not just for my enjoyment and fulfillment but for others who love and live differently from me to also relish it. And right now, that means getting our neighbors, our congregations and our communities of faith, our political world, to understand that prejudice and bigotry, racism and sexism, homophobia, transphobia, and heterosexism are not acceptable and will not be tolerated. May the Holy Spirit enliven us to turn the world upside down and inside out, to shape a world overflowing with love.

My hope for you is that you perceive yourself as wonderfully as God perceives you. And may the Spirit always guide you to take new risks... and to wear purple.

Wonder

When was the last time you walked by a building or bridge, a field, flower bed, forest, or a group of people and your breath was caught by the beauty of the view, the complexities of the scents you smelled, or the richness of the sounds you heard? Write about it. Compose a poem.

Share the experience with someone.

Ask someone to tell you about one of their "colorful" breathtaking experiences.

Resist

When was the last time you were challenged to observe and understand another person or community differently than you previously did?

How did that change your behaviors?

How can you learn about another person or community to reorient your perceptions or build understanding?

Embody

Is there anything in your story that weighs down your body, something the Spirit may be inviting you to release?

What feels light or what lightens your spirit? Add more of this to your routine!

Create

What color do you think of when you imagine yourself in your most carefree state of being? Why that color?

Create a space that integrates your color to be enlivened by it often.

Buy a piece of clothing in that color at a second-hand shop or store and go ahead and wear it!

Hope

What learning or wisdom have you gained in your life that has freed you from concerns about what others think of you?

Share that insight with someone who might benefit from it.

What aspiration do you have for the future? How can you "practice" for this now? How can you practice risk-tasking?

Stretch

Where in your life can you move out of the way so that another person who is different from you can have space to flourish?

What is keeping you from doing that right now?

How can you participate in turning the world "upside down and inside out"?

Share

Recall one or more "How else than by the Spirit" experiences. Tell someone about the Spirit at work in your life.

You have "care, wisdom, and love" to pass on to others. What gifts and graces do others see in you? Spend time discerning your gifts.

Share with someone your gratitude for how they have helped you see yourself and/or your gifts in new ways.

The Rainbow

Fearfully and Wonderfully Made

Marian Edmonds-Allen (she/they)

For it was you who formed my inward parts;
*   you knit me together in my mother's womb.*
I praise you, for I am fearfully and wonderfully made.
*   Wonderful are your works;*
*   that I know very well. (Psalm 139:13–14)*

You are fully known by God—after all, as the psalmist says, God formed your inmost self—and knit you together! And not only are you fully known, you are fully loved. In all your complexity, the many parts of you that comprise who you are. Like the colors of the rainbow flag, you are multifaceted and beautiful: "fearfully and wonderfully made."

I'm a rainbow myself, knit together with intersections that strengthen and complement each other. I'm blessed to direct Parity, an NYC-based national nonprofit that works in faith spaces to affirm LGBTQ+ people, and in LGBTQ+ places to affirm faith. We build bridges, most often trying to span divides that are filled with emotion—hurt and rejection—on both sides.

I joke that when I speak to a group, depending on the audience, I will scare someone. You see, I'm a queer pastor. For LGBTQ+ folks, hearing that I'm a person of faith usually sends ripples of dismay through the audience. And when I speak to audiences where faith is the focus and share that I am a gender diverse bisexual woman married to a woman, well, you can imagine the reaction that happens there! When I come "out" as either a person of faith or as a queer person, someone's world is rocked.

Like the colors of the Pride flag, my multiple identities are part of the beautiful whole that is the person I am—that *you* are—beautifully diverse, with each color making the others more vibrant and stronger. Each color radiates from each of us—but is illumined differently. Imagine the countless shades of any given color, the hues, tints, and intensity. Light. Bright. Subtle. Bold. Blended.

Not only are these colors revealed differently from person to person, but they are reflected in our lives uniquely from year to year...even day to day! Think again about each one:

Pink

Red

Orange

Yellow

Green

Turquoise

Blue

Purple

Recall Gilbert Baker's themes for each color; they too manifest differently in various seasons of our lives:

Sex

Life

Healing

Sunlight

Nature

Magic/Art

Harmony/Serenity

Spirit

I am reminded of the beautiful Nguni Bantu term *Ubuntu*, often translated "I am because we are" or "I am because you are." The rainbow colors and their meanings are richer in relationship with each other. Scholars have noted that the Trinity is relational within itself. God, Jesus, the Holy Spirit. Each of the three persons interacts with and enriches the other, and at the same time defines the other.

Ubuntu. A model for us as we seek to follow the triune God.

The rainbow. An illustration for us as we seek to honor ourselves and one another.

Our world has become (even) more divided of late. We can find more reasons to disagree than agree, even though we share much more in common than not. Worse still, our disagreements are rarely used to create or deepen relationships, but instead used to prevent new relationships or to destroy ties and bonds of friendship and love. Some people think about sin as not being in "right relationship" with God and with each other. I wonder if the sin of denying relationship with others has hardened our hearts so that we find it difficult to see and hear God in others, and as a result, to see and hear God reflected in our own selves.

I remember when I met my first openly LGBTQ+ person. I was working as a chaplain at a medical center, close to finishing my Master of Divinity degree, and very close to ordination. It had been a long process, seven years of full-time study coinciding with full-time work to support my four small children. I was a single mom, forty years old and pretty sure I had myself and the world figured out. Until I realized I didn't.

I was serving as a chaplain in a mental health unit, and four of my fellow chaplains were openly, proudly...LGBTQ+. I'll be honest, my world was rocked! Because of my sheltered background, I felt revulsion that I would need to associate with people "like that."

Well, I'm sure you can guess what happened next.

Yes, you know I'm LGBTQ+, so you guessed it. I saw that, like the story of the ugly duckling who realized she was a swan, I wasn't who I thought I was—at forty years old! I realized I was not a heterosexual person, but that I was a fabulous LGBTQ+ person. It didn't feel fabulous at the time.

At first, I was devastated.

I knew what the church said, "abomination!" and I thought I knew what God said, "God hates LGBTQ+ people!" I thought God hated me.

It was the worst timing for what I thought was the end of my life. Little did I know what would happen next.

I was about to graduate, about to be ordained. What was I to do? I went to my advisor at my theological school, a person I knew well and trusted. My advisor first argued with me, asserted that these were just false feelings. I wasn't really a lesbian (how I identified at that time). It was a phase, it would pass...My advisor and I disagreed about this, until finally in exasperation, they said, "Well, hide it, and if you are ever asked, just lie."

I thought about that. I thought about lying. I really did. I was SO close to graduating. Having devoted years to graduate school, navigating work and caring for my kids at the same time, I could just...pretend. But I knew I couldn't pretend, I couldn't lie.

I left that theological school, which did not then and does not now affirm LGBTQ+ people in leadership. I found my way back to God after months of study and learning about LGBTQ+ people of faith. I thought I was all alone. I thought there was no one like me. But that wasn't true.

Over 50 percent of LGBTQ+ people say they have some type of spirituality, faith, or religious belief. I just hadn't found my tribe. I wasn't alone at all, there were other rainbow swans out there. I also found books—oh, the books! AMAZING stories of LGBTQ+ faith journeys. I found books about how LGBTQ+ people read Scripture, I found something called queer theology. Who knew? As long as there have been people, there have been LGBTQ+ people and LGBTQ+ people of faith.

I now believe that queer people uniquely reflect God, and I believe that queer people of faith uniquely show the power of Christ's resurrection. Who else is told that by being who they are they can't follow Jesus? And yet, LGBTQ+ Christians not only follow Jesus but live and proclaim the gospel, showing the world a fuller understanding of who God is and how God loves us all.

I started at a new theological school, Eden Seminary, that specialized in progressive theology with affirming and LGBTQ+ professors. I found jobs at affirming churches, and after I graduated, I was recruited to Salt Lake City to start an LGBTQ+ affirming United Church of Christ church. My homeless youth ministry started there; everything I do today started there, a community of battered, bruised, yet hopeful LGBTQ+ people and allies, all searching to connect or reconnect with God.

We worshipped on Sunday and then brought hot food and supplies to about sixty LGBTQ+ youth living in camps around Salt Lake. And then I was asked to be the executive director of OUTreach Resource Center in Ogden, where we worked with 700 youth from three states, 30 percent of them experiencing homelessness, almost every one of them having lost someone they knew to suicide.

I was asked to not talk about faith with the youth at OUTreach or to talk about being an ordained clergyperson. Why? Because the board knew that religion hurts LGBTQ+ youth. I knew that, too, so I didn't talk about faith.

But what I discovered after a while is that even though I never mentioned God or faith, the LGBTQ+ youth I saw every week DID want to talk about both. They wanted to talk about God, about faith and spirituality, especially the youth experiencing homelessness. Every youth I met carried very little with them—how could they carry much? But one thing they carried was some type of journal to scribble thoughts, compose poems, or draw, *and to write to God*. One youth said, "Well, I've lost everything. I think God is all I have left."

We started a weekly spirituality group at OUTreach and invited LGBTQ+ people from all faiths to come and talk about their faith journeys, and we encouraged the youth to ask questions. Of all our activities, the spirituality discussion group was by far the most popular.

It wasn't about changing anyone's mind or changing anything. It was about holding space, what I call "grace space," to simply have a conversation about LGBTQ+ identities, experiences, and faith. Every perspective was not only welcome but sought. That's one of the most important things I've ever learned, to actively seek out new thoughts and ideas. I strive to do this every single day. For me, this is my faith in action. I believe that I learn more about God as I learn more about others, without limiting the people I interact with—that's key. The more different someone is, the more I am drawn to get to know them.

The challenge for me, and I wonder if you have a similar challenge, is to remain curious about all the rainbow parts of my own self. I made the mistake before of thinking I knew myself only to have my world upended. Part of my daily spiritual practice is to read Scripture, write, and simply notice who I am each day. It's hard to not be critical of myself but rather to pay attention and let Scripture illuminate what I notice as pathways to positive change and growth, within myself and in my relationships in the world. Devotionals like this one are important to me. Reading, reflecting, noticing pathways to positive change and growth. You know: wondering, resisting, embodying, creating, hoping, stretching, sharing.

Ubuntu. "I am because we are."

The rainbow. Each color enriching every other color.

My hope and prayer for you is that you celebrate yourself—all the parts knit together that make you the glorious reflection of God that you are. I also hope and pray that as you contemplate how God works in and through the lives of LGBTQ+ Christians, you find ways to invite the hurting, needy world into our allied world of resilience, strength, beauty, and love. LGBTQ+ people and allies have a way of living... embodying love, courage, and hope in a way that inspires others to be their authentic selves. It's a gift that God gave us, and it's a gift I invite you to share.

Who *you* are—your beautiful rainbow self of intertwining identities— you are a human bridge, fearfully and wonderfully made of the colors of hope. You are a bridge that connects people in ways that few can. You are blessed to be a blessing—*you.* LGBTQ+ you, ally you, curious questioning you. Discerning you. Faithful you. *All* of *you.* All of you, all of us. Thanks be to God.

Wonder

Write about how it feels to be "fearfully and wonderfully made," to be created and known so intimately by the God of all creation: the Creator, Redeemer and Sustainer.

Write about how it feels to honor everyone, to affirm that every body is fearfully and wonderfully made.

Resist

How do you resist the fading of your "rainbow colors"?

LGBTQ+ or not, what are your many identities that make you who you are?

What gives you energy and courage to shine as brightly as God intends you to shine?

Embody

Having engaged the many journal prompts throughout *Colors of Hope*, how will you embody your faith?

How will you "hope in color"?

How will you enrich the lives of others?

Create

Create a picture of your rainbow self, with words or as a drawing.

What colors + themes are the most vivid? Remember what they are: pink + sex, red + life, orange + healing, yellow + sunlight, green + nature, turquoise + magic/art, blue + harmony/serenity, and purple + spirit.

Hope

The author writes, "Who *you* are—your beautiful rainbow self of intertwining identities—you are a human bridge, fearfully and wonderfully made of the colors of hope. You are a bridge..." How are you a bridge? What are you bridging? With whom? Or how can you be a bridge?

If there is a divide in your life, filled with emotion—hurt and rejection or something else—*write to God.*

Identify someone you can talk with and/or use the resources at the conclusion of this book. You are not alone.

Stretch

Think about someone who is very different from you, someone who has different politics, perhaps, or different opinions on an issue you care about, or...

Write about what you would like to learn from them. What questions would you want them to answer?

What questions would you hope they ask you?

Share

The author says, "I was asked to not talk about faith with the youth at OUTreach or to talk about being an ordained clergyperson...Because the board knew that religion hurts LGBTQ+ youth." While it might be a stretch for you, talk about your faith journey. With one person or a group of people. Share questions that you have. Ask questions about their faith journeys.

Record parts of your faith journey here.

Finally, share *Colors of Hope*.

It is your turn to hope in color, imagining and shaping a brighter and more just future where the expansive love of God is embodied in every aspect of life.

Benediction

Hope.

Hope
in
color.

Called by name, our rainbow selves are celebrated:
Beloved
Child of God
"This is who I am!"
This is who we are.

Called to name every body,
to embrace every body,
to affirm every body:
every body fearfully and wonderfully made
of the colors of hope.

Called:
to wonder
resist
embody

create

hope

stretch

and share.

We are sent out to transform narratives of injustice

and write the next chapters of liberation.

Wave the flags, paint your faces, paint the world,

dance, sing, raise a glass, (safely) join in parades and protests.

Proclaiming (rarely with words), "This is who we are!"

Go

with joy

in peace

empowered,

with Pride.

Amen. And amen. And amen.

About AllianceQ –
the Disciples LGBTQ+ Alliance

AllianceQ – the Disciples LGBTQ+ Alliance is more than forty years old, with its beginnings in 1979 as GLAD: the Gay, Lesbian and Affirming Disciples Alliance. Our ministry supports lesbian, gay, bisexual, transgender, and gender-diverse people of faith. We educate and equip faith communities for understanding, affirming, and including LGBTQ+ persons, and we collaborate with ecumenical partners for intersectional justice work.

AllianceQ advocates alongside LGBTQ+ organizations to urge nondiscrimination and address queer issues. We aim to elevate the voices of affirming faith leaders to change the social landscape. The Alliance engages in ongoing anti-racism work, seeking to bridge the gap between racial, ethnic, gender and sexual diversity as movements for racial justice and LGBTQ+ liberation are deeply intertwined with interconnected histories.

We are members of the Body of Christ, called to join in God's work of transforming the Christian Church (Disciples of Christ) into a just and inclusive church that welcomes persons of all gender identities and expressions and sexual orientations into full life and leadership of the church.

The Christian Church (Disciples of Christ) recognizes the changing context of congregational life and ministry and is seeking a wider embrace of persons of all gender expressions and sexual identities. The 2013 General Assembly meeting in Orlando, Florida, passed a resolution stating that the Church welcomes all, and for the first time, included sexual orientation as an identity that should not be denied the radical welcome of Christ and Christ's church.[12] The 2019 General Assembly meeting in Des Moines, Iowa, passed a resolution

---

[12]GA-1327, Becoming a People of Grace and Welcome to All.

inviting the whole church to educate itself about transgender and gender-diverse persons.[13] In a joint reflection of faith from General Minister and President Terri Hord Owens and AllianceQ Executive Director + Minister Melissa Guthrie in January 2020, Rev. Hord Owens emphasized: "We cannot mandate adherence to either resolution, but with the leadership of many regions, clergy and congregations, as well as ministries such as Disciples AllianceQ, we can offer the space for discernment and education as we all seek to follow the command of Christ to love each one whom God has created."[14]

The Alliance uses LGBTQ+ for an expansive community represented by a range of initialisms. We acknowledge that language and identity are constantly evolving. Our ministry continues to evolve:

It was at the 1977 General Assembly in Kansas City, Missouri, that the late Carol Blakely of Caldwell, Idaho, a Disciple mother of a gay son, broke silence and called all Disciples to name the reality that LGBTQ+ and affirming persons are our sons, daughters, brothers, sisters, parents, congregants, pastors and staff.

Sparked by that moment, a small group of gay and lesbian Disciples began to coalesce. The first—secret—meeting was held at the St. Louis, Missouri, General Assembly in 1979. The meeting was held away from the Assembly site and those who gathered only used first names. For eight years, meetings continued. The first newsletter, *Crossbeams*, emerged in January 1987, edited by Allen V. Harris (author of "How else than by the Spirit," the reflection on purple + spirit in this devotional!). At a pre-assembly event in October 1987, in Louisville, Kentucky, the organization was named: the Gay, Lesbian, and Affirming Disciples Alliance.

Always an "alliance" (check out the definition), the organization expanded. The name was bold and daring in 1987, but less inclusive than the mission and ministry pursued. The organization sought a title that intentionally named the four aspects of our community that have historically joined together: L, G, B, and T. And a title that left room for growth. Leaders adopted "The Disciples LGBTQ+ Alliance" in 2017.

---

[13]GA-1929, An Invitation to Education for Welcoming and Receiving the Gifts of Transgender and Gender-Diverse People.

[14]"No one excluded from God's love," Christian Church (Disciples of Christ), January 2020. https://disciples.org/from-the-gmp/no-one-excluded-from-gods-love/.

The identity statement of the Christian Church (Disciples of Christ) states: "We are Disciples of Christ, a movement for wholeness in a fragmented world. As part of the one body of Christ we welcome all to the Lord's Table as God has welcomed us."[15] And so we celebrate our identity as Disciples.

Q claims our pride in the face of oppression and Q includes those who do not claim the binaries or boxes of L, G, B, and T.

+ reminds us that there will always be yet another neighbor to include.

+ reminds us that we cannot do our ministry without affirming friends and allies.

+ reminds us that we cannot do our ministry without the individuals and groups who also find themselves in the margins.

AllianceQ is our moniker. We are a member-based organization and invite you to be part of our movement for wholeness. There is a place for you at the Table.

---

[15]"Our Identity Statement," Christian Church (Disciples of Christ), https://disciples.org/our-identity/.

Resources

Your Neighbors

Intentional relationships with others will always be the greatest opportunity for us to learn about ourselves, others, and the world.

AllianceQ

With more than 300 resources, the Alliance can support you on your journey and connect you with other people of faith. Find an Open & Affirming ministry, become an Open & Affirming ministry, learn, *connect.*
disciplesallianceq.org

The Christian Church (Disciples of Christ)

Christian Church (Disciples of Christ)
disciples.org

Disciples Justice Ministries
disciples.org/resources/justice

The National Benevolent Association (NBA)
The health and social services general ministry of the Christian Church (Disciples of Christ).
nbacares.org

LGBTQ+ History and the Pride Flag

The LGBTQ Religious Archives Network (LGBTQ-RAN)
lgbtqreligiousarchives.org

The GLBT Historical Society
glbthistory.org

The Gilbert Baker Foundation
gilbertbaker.com

Mental Health and Wellness

It Gets Better Project
Inspiring stories from LGBTQ+ youth and adults.
itgetsbetter.org

The Trevor Project
Leading national organization providing crisis intervention and suicide prevention services to LGBTQ young people under 25. The TrevorLifeline is 866-488-7386.
thetrevorproject.org

Trans Lifeline
Provides trans peer support for our community that's been divested from police. Call 877-565-8860.
translifeline.org

Welcoming and Affirming Ministries

AllianceQ – the Disciples LGBTQ+ Alliance
disciplesallianceq.org

Association of Welcoming & Affirming Baptists (AWAB)
awab.org

Brethren Mennonite Council for LGBT Interest
bmclgbt.org

Extraordinary Lutheran Ministries
elm.org

The Fellowship of Affirming Ministries (TFAM)
radicallyinclusive.org

Institute for Welcoming Resources
welcomingresources.org

Many Voices
manyvoices.org

Metropolitan Community Churches
mcchurch.org

More Light Presbyterians
mlp.org

Open and Affirming Coalition of the United Church of Christ
openandaffirming.org

Parity
parity.nyc

Q Christian Fellowship
qchristian.org

Reconciling Ministries Network (RMN)
rmnetwork.org

ReconcilingWorks
reconcilingworks.org

The Reformation Project
reformationproject.org

Room for All (RfA)
roomforall.com

TransFaith
transfaith.info

Unitarian Universalist Association
uua.org

General LGBTQ+ Organizations and Resources

GLAAD
GLAAD counters discrimination against LGBTQ individuals in the
media and promotes understanding, acceptance, and equality.
glaad.org

GLSEN
Works to ensure that LGBTQ students can learn and grow in a school
environment free from bullying and harassment.
glsen.org

My Pronouns
mypronouns.org

The Naming Project
Provides a safe place for LGBTQ+ youth to grow and discuss faith and
equips those who care for LGBTQ+ youth.
thenamingproject.org/about

National Center for Transgender Equality (NCTE)
Resources, self-help guides, info about transgender people.
transequality.org

National LGBTQ Task Force
Advocacy opportunities and news.
thetaskforce.org

PFLAG
Support, education, and advocacy to LGBTQ+ people, their parents
and families, and allies.
pflag.org

Practice with Pronouns
practicewithpronouns.com

Candace Chellew-Hodge, *Bulletproof Faith: A Spiritual Survival Guide
for Gay and Lesbian Christians* (Hoboken, NJ: Wiley, 2008).

Matthew Vines, *God and the Gay Christian: The Biblical Case in Support
of Same-Sex Relationships* (New York: Convergent Books, 2015).

Ross Murray, *Made, Known, Loved: Developing LGBTQ-Inclusive Youth
Ministry* (Minneapolis, MN: Fortress Press, 2021).

Mihee Kim-Kort, *Outside the Lines: How Embracing Queerness Will
Transform Your Faith* (Minneapolis, MN: Fortress Press, 2018).

Leigh Finke, *Queerfully and Wonderfully Made: A Guide for LGBTQ+ Christian Teens* (Minneapolis, MN: Beaming Books, 2020).

Austen Hartke, *Transforming: The Bible and the Lives of Transgender Christians* (Louisville, KY: Westminster John Knox Press, 2017).

Brandan Robertson, *True Inclusion: Creating Communities of Radical Embrace* (St. Louis, MO: Chalice Press, 2018).

Leigh Finke, *Welcoming and Affirming: A Guide to Supporting and Working with LGBTQ+ Christian Youth* (Minneapolis, MN: Broadleaf Books, 2020).

Organization descriptions adopted from their websites.

About the Editor

Rev. Melissa Lynn Guthrie (she/her) is the Executive Director + Minister with AllianceQ – the Disciples LGBTQ+ Alliance and the founding director of Salvage Garden. She created "The Banquet: A Sensory Worship Experience," centering disabled individuals. Melissa is trained in faith-based nonprofit leadership through Wake Forest University Divinity and Law Schools. A lecturer on theology and disability, she is passionate about the many intersections of our identities. Among her identities, Melissa is a minister, ordained by the Christian Church (Disciples of Christ), and mother. Melissa and her wife Leah live in Greensboro, North Carolina, with their children and a small zoo.

The Iowa native studied Communications and Religion at Wartburg College and received Youth and Family Ministry Certification from Wartburg Seminary. The Spirit moved Melissa to North Carolina to teach high school English as a corps member with Teach for America. Melissa then pursued her Master of Divinity from Wake Forest University School of Divinity. She enjoys cheesecake and cycling, in that order. Melissa likes being outdoors and reading and writing poetry (outdoors). Pink and yellow are her favorite colors.